Contents

Natural Remedies
for
Dogs and Cats

Natural Remedies *for* Dogs and Cats

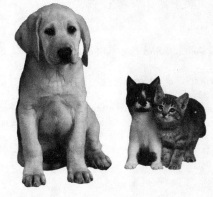

CJ Puotinen

KEATS PUBLISHING

LOS ANGELES

NTC/Contemporary Publishing Group

Natural Remedies for Dogs and Cats is not intended as medical advice. Its intent is solely informational and educational. Please consult a health professional should the need for one be indicated.

Library of Congress Cataloging-in-Publication Data

Puotinen, CJ
   Natural Remedies for Dogs and Cats/CJ Puotinen.
       p.   cm.
   Includes bibliographical references (p.   ) and index.
   ISBN 0-87983-827-2
   1. Dogs—Diseases—Alternative treatment.   2. Cats—Diseases—
   Alternative treatment.   3. Dogs—Health.   4. Cats—Health
   5. Holistic veterinary medicine.   I. Title
   SF991.P86   1999   99-26191
   636.7'0893—dc21   CIP

Interior design: Cheryl Carrington

Published by Keats Publishing
A division of NTC/Contemporary Publishing Group, Inc.
4255 West Touhy Avenue, Lincolnwood, Illinois 60646-1975 U.S.A.

Printed in the United States of America

International Standard Book Number: 0-87983-827-2

99 00 01 02 03 04 DHD 18 17 16 15 14 13 12 11 10 9 8 7 6 5 4 3 2 1

To the memory of *Kanga*

(June 18, 1967–July 11, 1987)

and her daughter, *Hang Twelve*

(July 23, 1968–February 14, 1988),

the smartest and sweetest cats who ever lived,

and to *Pumpkin*

(May 15, 1990–June 12, 1993),

a bold, friendly spirit who left too soon

Introduction

I n our age of modern medicine, when illnesses are treated in high-tech hospitals with laser surgery and powerful prescription drugs, it is easy to forget that until the twentieth century, herbs and food were the medicines that kept people and their companion animals well. Most of the prescription drugs in use today are derived and synthesized from plants, and in most parts of the world, plants are still the primary healing agents.

The surgical techniques and pharmaceutical drugs that define Western medicine work well in acute or crisis conditions, but they are far less successful in the treatment of chronic illnesses. Western medicine, as practiced by physicians and veterinarians, is allopathic, which means that its focus is on the alleviation or suppression of physical symptoms, not on the treatment of the causes of these symptoms. Chronic conditions such as arthritis, skin and coat problems, gingivitis, ear infections, asthma, and allergies may improve temporarily when their symptoms are masked, but they usually recur and, over time, grow worse. For this reason, conventional or orthodox medicine considers these conditions irreversible and incurable. In addition, the drugs and surgery used to treat them carry adverse side effects that range from minor to fatal.

The advantage of natural remedies is that they often work as well as or better than conventional treatments, have fewer side effects, and address the cause of a condition, resulting in its improvement or cure. Because of the limitations of allopathic medicine, many Americans have turned to natural approaches to health and healing. Natural therapies do not improve every condition in every person or pet, but they offer a first line of defense in the prevention of problems and, when an illness is well established, can help speed healing.

Natural Remedies for Dogs and Cats offers a holistic approach to feeding and enhancing the health of your pet that can help your dog or cat live longer, heal faster, stay flexible, and enjoy good health through an active old age. My previous book, *The Encyclopedia of Natural Pet Care* (also available from Keats Publishing), contains more detailed instructions for using herbs, homeopathy, aromatherapy, natural light, color, hands-on therapies, flower essences, nutritional supplements and other holistic healing methods. I hope you will consult *The Encyclopedia of Natural Pet Care* if you need more comprehensive instructions than can be included here.

An informed owner is a pet's best medical insurance. Keep on hand not only this book but also others recommended in these pages, for each offers a different perspective. I am not a veterinarian, scientist, health care worker, breeder, trainer, groomer, or pet store owner or employee, nor do I make or sell pet-related products. Although I have studied and written about medicinal plants, I am not a practicing herbalist. I have no financial interest in any of the products, services, or procedures recommended here. My perspective is that of a writer who lives with and loves animals. In order to learn what I wanted to know, I read everything I could find and interviewed every expert who would speak with me.

In the field of holistic pet care, these experts are not only well informed and articulate, they're also very nice people. I owe special thanks to pet nutritionists Marina Zacharias, Pat McKay, Celeste Yarnall, Bea Lydecker, and Kymythy Schultze; to herbalists Jean Argus, Deb Soule, Ed Smith, and James Green; to aromatherapists Suzanne Catty, Kristen Leigh Bell, and Patricia Whitaker; to many responsible breeders who feed their dogs and cats raw foods, including Sarah Wilson Kilcommons, Joan Andreasen-Webb, Barbara Werner, Nancy Strouss, Diane Laratta, Darla Duffey, Christine Swingle, Kathy Herman, Jo Forsythe, and Cathy Winkler, for sharing with me their experiences, knowledge, and expertise; and to Nancy Kern, editor of *The Whole Dog Journal*, which has published my articles on canine nutrition and herbs, portions of which are included in this book.

In addition, my gratitude goes to Phyllis Herman, my editor at Keats Publishing, for her guidance and good sense; to my teacher, Rosemary Gladstar, for introducing me to the history and use of medicinal herbs; to Dora Gerber, owner of the Swissette Herb Farm in Salisbury Mills, New York, who gave me practical experience and taught me the herbal traditions of her native Switzerland and Western Europe; to my husband, Joel Hollenberg, for his encouragement and support; and to Samantha (black Labrador Retriever), Pepper (black cat), and Pumpkin II (red tabby kitten), who make our house a home.

Because I want *Natural Remedies for Dogs and Cats* to be a useful tool, I have included as many resources as possible at the back of this book, with names, addresses, phone numbers, fax numbers, E-mail addresses, and Web sites. To find a company that has moved since this book went to press, check current issues of pet magazines, the referral services of national organizations, newsletter editors, or public library reference desks.

Please keep in mind that my purpose is to define, explain, and demonstrate herbal and nutritional techniques that many pet owners have used with good results. Nothing in this book is meant to diagnose a specific illness or prescribe a specific treatment for your pet. No alternative or complementary treatment is a cure-all that will work in every case or for every animal. However, the more knowledgeable you are about your pet and its species, the more you understand its digestive processes and nutritional requirements, and the more you learn about common illnesses and how to prevent them, the happier, healthier, and longer your animal's life is likely to be.

Readers are invited to send their experiences, comments, and discoveries pertaining to herbs and natural health for dogs and cats to me at the address below. For a reply, please enclose a stamped, self-addressed business-size envelope. Write to:

CJ Puotinen
P. O. Box 525
Hoboken, NJ 07030-0525

Chapter 1

Feeding Your Pet the Right Way

In the United States, most of us think that "people food" should not be given to dogs or cats. For half a century, pet food manufacturers and veterinarians have convinced us that because commercial foods are designed in laboratories by people with academic credentials and because their labels contain long lists of nutrients and claims of being "scientifically balanced" and "nutritionally complete," they are superior to anything our animals might otherwise consume. Table scraps, raw food, human food, and supplements that might disrupt commercial food's precisely controlled distribution of vitamins and minerals are particularly frowned on.

We're so used to these notions that most of us accept them without a second thought. But all along, some pet owners have taken a different approach, and in recent years their murmur of protest has become a rallying cry.

What are these eccentric people feeding their pets? Just the things that the experts say will kill them: home-prepared human foods, fruits and vegetables, raw meat, unpasteurized milk, raw eggs, and—worst of all—raw bones. If their dogs and cats don't die from indigestion, botulism,

Salmonella, E. coli, or a deficiency disease, they'll surely choke to death or puncture their intestines. Any veterinarian will tell you that these animals are living on borrowed time.

Make that almost any veterinarian. Members of the American Holistic Veterinary Medical Association, an organization that reflects the surging interest in natural therapies, believe those animals are eating exactly what Mother Nature intended. While writing *The Encyclopedia of Natural Pet Care,* I interviewed holistic veterinarians and animal health care professionals nationwide. When I asked them about specific illnesses, they offered many different therapies, for each had a different approach to health and healing. But when I asked them why America's pets have so many problems, each blamed the same two factors. "Commercial pet foods," they all said, "and annual vaccinations. That's why our pets are so sick."

The debate over pet foods is ongoing, from the source and quality of their ingredients to their use of chemical preservatives, colors, and flavoring agents. Only a few premium brands contain foods suitable for consumption by humans; almost all are made from such questionable raw materials that they have been the subject of lengthy exposés by veterinarians and investigative journalists.

The meat and other ingredients used in pet foods, their large proportion of grains, the safety of widely used preservatives, and the end result's digestibility and nutritional balance are serious concerns, but according to a growing number of experts, none of these is the most important issue. For that, they say, we must consider an experiment conducted half a century ago at a human health clinic in California.

The Pottenger Cat Study

In 1932, Francis M. Pottenger Jr., M.D., was a mainstream physician, author of medical journal articles, and president of the Los Angeles County Medical Association. Dr. Pottenger noticed that the health of his clinic's resident cats, which appeared to be well fed on a diet of raw milk, cod liver oil, and cooked meat scraps, had in fact declined. This observation inspired him to embark on a ten-year study conducted according to the most rigorous scientific standards of the day, during which 900 cats were studied and complete records were kept on 600.

All of the cats were fed scraps of the meat served at the sanatorium, which included beef, lamb, and poultry muscle meats; bones; and organs such as liver, tripe, sweetbreads (the pancreas and/or thymus), brain, and heart. All of the meat was organically raised and of the highest quality.

The cats were housed in large outdoor pens near a stand of eucalyptus trees on the side of a hill overlooking the San Gabriel Valley. Each pen had an open-air enclosure 12 feet long, 6 feet wide, and 7 feet high screened with chicken wire so the cats had adequate sun exposure. A trench 18 inches deep was dug inside the enclosure and filled with freshly washed sand. The cats were protected from inclement weather by a roofed area with a wooden floor and bedding material. A caretaker removed bones and uneaten food daily, and cleaned and refilled the water containers. Periodically, he removed the cats' buried excreta from the sand for composting in piles labeled according to the cats' diets.

The cats were fed a diet of two-thirds meat, one-third milk, and small amounts of cod liver oil. One group received both raw meat and raw milk, and this was the only group to reproduce generation after generation of healthy kittens with broad faces, adequate nasal cavities, broad dental arches, strong and correctly shaped teeth and bones, excellent tissue tone, good quality fur with a minimum of shedding, and an absence of gum disease. These cats were resistant to infections, fleas, and internal parasites. They showed no sign of allergies and were gregarious, friendly, and predictable in their behavior patterns. Miscarriages were rare, and litters averaged five kittens, which the mothers nursed without difficulty. Some cats received raw meat and pasteurized milk, others received cooked meat and raw milk, and some received canned, condensed, or sweetened condensed milk with raw meat. None was fed everything cooked: they all had either raw milk or raw meat with the other portion of their diet cooked or pasteurized. All of the cats in these groups suffered from nutritional deficiencies.

The cats fed cooked meat developed skeletal and dental deformities; heart and vision problems; thyroid imbalances; infections of the kidney, liver, testes, ovaries, and bladder; arthritis and inflammation of the joints; and inflammation of the nervous system with paralysis and meningitis. Their second and third generations had abnormal respiratory tissues. Female cooked-meat cats were so irritable that some were named Tiger, Cobra, and Rattlesnake, while the males were docile and passive, a sexual role reversal not seen in the raw-food cats. Vermin and intestinal parasites abounded, skin lesions and allergies appeared frequently, and adult cats died of pneumonia or infections of the bone while kittens died of pneumonia and diarrhea. The cooked-meat cats had serious reproductive problems, including sterility, miscarriage, lack of maternal instinct, and difficult labors with high infant mortality rates. Many females died in labor.

The cats fed raw meat with pasteurized milk showed similar changes, and those fed evaporated milk showed even more damage, while the most marked deficiencies occurred among those fed sweetened condensed milk.

Because the health of each new generation was adversely affected by its parents' inferior diet, the cooked-food kittens had even more problems, and there were no fourth-generation kittens in the cooked-food groups because the third generation died before reproducing. Had antibiotic drugs been available, these kittens might not have died of pneumonia and other infectious diseases, in which case the experiment could have continued through longer chains of deformed offspring.

One of Pottenger's most exciting discoveries was that the health deterioration caused by cooked foods could be reversed, although it took four generations to completely restore to perfect health those cats whose predecessors consumed cooked meat or pasteurized milk.

As Pottenger demonstrated, our pets have problems because their parents and grandparents ate cooked food, and these problems increase as a result of the cooked food they consume. By changing from cooked to raw foods, an animal's health may improve even though its skeleton and teeth will not be transformed.

Although his cat experiment was the largest and most ambitious, Pottenger also studied the effects of cooked or heated food on other animals, including guinea pigs, chickens, and cattle. In every case, he found that the absence of raw food, or what he called fresh factors, made the difference between perfect health and serious illness.

The Pottenger cat study is thoroughly documented in the book *Pottenger's Cats*, published by the Price-Pottenger Nutrition Foundation. According to editor Elaine Pottenger in the book's introduction, the experiment is often misrepresented. She explains, "One author of a popular book states that 200 cats died of arthritis. Indeed, this did not happen. Another author states that the cats were fed sprouts and survived in full health for four continuous generations. Again, no such experiment took place, and yet this misinformation has been reported in over a dozen or more different articles and books."

Perhaps the most widespread misrepresentation of the study is that the cooked-food cats received both cooked meat and pasteurized milk, a distortion that has encouraged many to conclude that feeding at least some raw food improves an animal's health. Although this may be true, nothing in the experiment supports that conclusion, for Pottenger's unhealthy cats received raw meat with their pasteurized milk or raw milk with their cooked meat.

Pottenger was not the only scientist to test the difference that cooking makes. When Sir Robert McCarrison fed monkeys in India their usual diet cooked instead of raw, the animals developed colitis. Their autopsies revealed gastric and intestinal ulcers. O. Stiner in Switzerland cooked the food his healthy guinea pigs had been eating raw; they developed anemia, scurvy, goiter, dental cavities, and malfunctions of the salivary glands. They developed arthritis as well after pasteurized milk was added to their daily fare.

When cooked food is fed to lions, tigers, and other predators in zoos, their health deteriorates. These animals prefer fresh raw food to anything that has been frozen and thawed, and they prefer wild game to meat that was domestically raised. Dogs and cats have the same instinctive preferences, which is why they respond so dramatically to freshly captured wild prey, fresh venison, and other free-range fare.

In attempting to duplicate Mother Nature, pet owners must consider where and how their pets' foods are raised. Most of the meat, poultry, eggs, and milk available in the United States is produced from animals that are fed and housed very differently from their counterparts on organic or biodynamic farms. As this book goes to press in the summer of 1999, the U.S. Department of Agriculture is, amid much controversy, developing a national standard for organically grown produce and organically raised animal products. Labeling is already confusing because lawsuits and lobbying efforts by pharmaceutical companies and irradiation equipment manufacturers have made it difficult or illegal for manufacturers to indicate on labels that their products are not made from genetically engineered plants or from milk that contains synthetic growth hormones, or that they have not been irradiated. Now the term *organic* is being redefined. Health magazines and organic gardening publications and bulletins posted in health food stores will help you remain an informed consumer.

The Best Diet for Dogs and Cats

What should dogs and cats eat? Everything about their anatomy points to a meat-based diet. Like the fox, coyote, wolf, hyena, lion, tiger, and other wild relatives, domestic dogs and cats have sharp teeth for tearing flesh and gnawing on bones, their digestive secretions are highly concentrated, and their intestines are short, all of which makes them well suited for processing freshly killed animals. Ruminants and humans, on the other hand, have flat molars for grinding grain or fibrous plants, and long digestive tracts that absorb the slowly released nutrients those foods contain.

At the same time, unlike Pottenger's cats, dogs are not true carnivores. From biblical times and earlier, canines around the world have been known as scavengers and omnivores. Left to their own devices, they eat a constantly changing variety of plants and animals, deriving calories and nutrients from meat, bones, the contents of their prey's digestive organs, and whatever fruits, vegetables, grasses, roots, eggs, berries, manure, and other edibles they can find.

While England and Europe were developing commercial pet foods in the 1940s and 1950s, Juliette de Bairacli Levy fed her unvaccinated Afghan Hounds raw meat, raw bones, raw goat's milk, raw fish, raw eggs, and a variety of raw fruits, vegetables, nuts, and oils. The only medicines she used were herbs. Supremely healthy and intelligent, her dogs won numerous championships. De Bairacli Levy, who described her Natural Rearing philosophy in a series of books, gained a devoted following around the world.

"Many people are doing a natural food diet nowadays," says Jo Forsythe, a longtime Newfoundland fancier who now breeds Portuguese Water Dogs, "but Juliette de Bairacli Levy deserves credit as the grandmother of the movement. I have friends who have followed her guidelines exclusively for many, many generations of healthy dogs. For convenience, I've had to modify her plan when I travel, but at home my dogs eat an almost all-raw diet. They don't have digestive problems or deficiency diseases, and they thrive on fresh, whole foods. I think that by eating a constantly changing assortment of foods, they have a better chance of getting whatever nutrients they need than if they ate the same foods every day."

Pet nutritionist Pat McKay, whose book *Reigning Cats and Dogs* has helped many make the transition from commercial pet foods to a home-prepared diet, agrees. "The easiest way to have a healthy pet," she says, "is to feed a variety of raw foods, the key words being *raw* and *variety*."

Early in his practice, Australian veterinarian Ian Billinghurst read American and English veterinary journals with wonder, for they routinely featured articles about illnesses and conditions he had never seen. In his book *Give Your Dog a Bone*, Billinghurst describes what happened when his nation adopted commercial pet foods in the 1960s. Until then, Australians fed their pets raw bones and table scraps. "Everybody knew how to do it," he says. "It was common sense. As a consequence, most Australian dogs were very healthy."

Billinghurst fed his own dogs commercial food for two years and watched them develop skin problems, runny eyes, scruffy coats, itching skin, hot spots, ear infections, anal sac problems, smelly fur and feces, bad breath, tooth and gum problems, repeated worm infestations, bone and growth disorders, and reproductive problems. Previously, his dogs had dined on fresh hare, raw bones, and table scraps. They were never wormed or vaccinated, had large litters of robust puppies, and stayed healthy with a minimum of effort.

As soon as Billinghurst switched his dogs back to their previous diet, their health improved. So did the health of dogs belonging to clients who adopted his feeding plan, and now, thanks to his books, speaking tours, and the success of his BARF (Bones And Raw Food or Biologically Appropriate Raw Food) philosophy, so has the health of dogs around the world.

Now, increasing numbers of American dog and cat breeders and owners are making their own comparisons. Marina Zacharias saw the difference when she bought her first Basset Hound fourteen years ago. "He had been raised on a premium-quality pet food for the first five and a half months of his life," she says. "I switched him over to a raw-food diet, which he had a much easier time digesting, and he grew very well. When he was eighteen months old, I saw some of his littermates, and the contrast was amazing. He had been one of the smaller puppies in the litter, and now he was the largest. His coat, bone density, posture, eyes, disposition, alertness, and everything else were superior."

Her first dog became the patriarch of a line of raw-food Bassets, and Zacharias became a full-time animal nutritionist and publisher of the *Natural Rearing* newsletter. "It works the other way around, too," she continues. "I know breeders who raised their puppies on raw food and sent them to show homes where for one reason or another their diet was changed. When they met up with the pups in show-handling class a few months later, their coat quality and bone density had deteriorated and they didn't look as well as they used to. It's not that a raw-food diet pushes growth, which would be unhealthy, but it meets the animal's genetic potential by providing all the nutrients the body needs to grow properly." Breeders who feed a natural diet do more than strengthen individual dogs; they improve their entire line. Barbara Werner raises Golden Retrievers in New Jersey. "When we had our first puppies from a four-year-old mother who has been on raw food all her life," she told me, "the difference was dramatic. She showed none of the signs of nutritional stress that are common in pregnancy. Her coat stayed gorgeous, her labor was short, and she produced nine strong, lively pups that landed on their feet. This is a breed so prone to autoimmune disorders and cancers that one veterinarian told me a three-year-old Golden is now considered middle-aged. I find this attitude unacceptable. The puppies' eleven-year-old grandfather is still so vibrant, he wins ribbons at dog shows."

Raw-food diets are intimidating to the uninitiated not because they are difficult to prepare but because they are unfamiliar. "Don't forget that we have all been brainwashed to believe that dogs should eat processed dog food and that raw bones are bad," says Christine Swingle, who raises West Highland White Terriers in Connecticut. "I have been feeding a raw-food diet for four years, and last year I gathered up the courage to feed raw chicken necks and wings. The Westies love them. It's amazing—they digest raw meaty bones despite what I was led to believe!"

Kymythy Schultze, an animal health instructor and author of *The Ultimate Diet*, has raised Newfoundlands for twenty years. "Natural health is today's hot topic," she says, "but I like to remind people that when we adopt a raw diet and use natural therapies, we're not doing anything new. We're doing something old-fashioned. When I made the transition eleven years ago, I met Newfie breeders who were still feeding their dogs the way everyone did before commercial pet foods were developed. These dogs ate the same raw meat, raw bones, and table scraps that people had been feeding their dogs for thousands of years, and they were strong and healthy, with calm dispositions, terrific coats, a resistance to fleas, and a total absence of doggy odors."

Kathy Herman realized the benefits of raw food when she visited Labrador Retriever breeders in England and for the first time met supremely healthy dogs. On a diet of raw bones, raw meat, raw goat's milk, vegetable peelings and other table scraps, and cereal-based kibble, these minimally vaccinated dogs suffered from none of the problems common to American Labs. Herman adopted a similar regimen and gradually reduced the amount of kibble until her dogs were eating all raw food. Since she improved their diet fifteen years ago, her dogs have been free of orthopedic problems, and the only puppies whose owners reported health problems were those who switched back to commercial food.

"My puppies go to people who are motivated and informed," she says, "and I give them a three-day supply of raw food to help them get used to its preparation. I didn't put raw foods into my contract until three years ago, when the owners of an eight-month-old female called to say she was limping and the specialist recommended immediate surgery. When I asked if they were still feeding raw food, they said their veterinarian had frightened them into feeding one of the dog foods he sold at his clinic because raw meat is dangerous and raw chicken bones would make her sick."

After Herman convinced the owners to resume a natural diet, the dog made a rapid recovery without surgery or prescription drugs. "Most veterinarians know very little about nutrition," she says, "but because they are authority figures, they can be intimidating. They recommend commercial pet foods because they don't have experience with anything else."

Darla Duffey, who bred Shetland Sheepdogs on raw food for many years, uses a natural diet to improve the health of homeless dogs that come to her through the adoption agency Sheltie Rescue. "We try to place our rescued Shelties with people who have lost a dog to cancer, lupus, kidney disease, or one of the other illnesses common in this breed," she explains. "I tell them that if they don't want the problem to happen again soon, they've got to keep the dog on a healthy diet. I go into the whys and wherefores, and in most cases, the lightbulb goes on in their head as they make the connection.

"Here in Florida we have a terrible flea problem," she adds, "but as soon as they go on raw foods, our rescued Shelties stop itching, their skin heals, their coats improve, and they're less attractive to fleas. They look more alert, they're less anxious, and their eyes are bright. This breed's health has been going down the tubes for a long time and it's going to take several generations to get it back on the right track. Fortunately, it doesn't take long to improve the health of individual dogs."

Cat breeders and owners who have made the transition to raw foods make the same claims. Their cats have healthier coats, better teeth, stronger bones, fewer respiratory infections, fewer urinary tract infections, and fewer problems with fleas and internal parasites as a result.

Learning to Feed Like Mother Nature

Food is one part of natural feeding. The timing of meals is another. Animals in the wild don't spend all day lounging around food dispensers; their digestive systems are stimulated only when food is available. Wild predators hunt when they're hungry. They may not find a substantial meal for hours or days, and when they do, they eat their fill. If there's nothing left over when they feel hungry, they hunt again. Dogs and cats evolved on a cycle of feasting and fasting, and as a result their digestive organs are designed to deal with large quantities of food followed by long periods during which the digestive tract empties and rests.

Proponents of raw, natural diets for dogs and cats recommend creating a modified version of this feeding cycle. In addition to removing food between meals and feeding adults only once or twice per day, they recommend letting the animal fast one day per week. Fasting means no food, only water. Although it's easier for young animals to adapt to this schedule, healthy dogs and cats of all ages adjust, and the next day they usually are more attentive, alert, affectionate, responsive, and focused. Most people assume that's because they're starving, but it's because the fast leaves them feeling better and more like their true selves instead of cranky, logy, heavy, dull, sluggish, and out of sorts from constant feeding.

Fasting is such a radical notion to some that it generates much confusion and anxiety. After all, food is love, and if I don't feed them, I'm negligent or abusive and they won't love me any more or they'll stare at me all night with big, sad, brown eyes and I'll feel awful. Human cultural conditioning has nothing to do with the nutritional needs of dogs and cats. Fasting requires the application of common sense—you should not, for example, fast a puppy, kitten, very small pet (miniature or toy breed), or any animal in fragile health for more than half a day. In combination with a well-balanced, natural, raw diet, healthy dogs and cats thrive on a fasting cycle, which improves the appetite, gives digestive organs a well-deserved rest, clears the intestinal tract, helps remove toxins from the body, improves the quality of sleep, and stimulates the production of digestive secretions for improved assimilation when food is presented.

Before adopting a fast-day feeding cycle, see pages 94–98 and 203–208 for important information about the detoxification process and its nutritional support. Detoxification is a constant process in all living creatures; it is the body's way of eliminating everything it doesn't need. A raw, bone-based diet with a few key supplements provides the nutrition dogs and cats need for the effective removal of stored toxins.

How Much Meat?

It is impossible to recommend a specific amount that will apply to every dog and cat because animals are as different from one another as people are. Is your animal large or small? Active or sedentary? Growing or mature? Wiry or portly? Living in a cold climate or in the tropics? In general, active working dogs, lively adolescent cats, and pets with a fast metabolism need more food than their sedentary or elderly relatives, and animals that spend considerable time outdoors need more food in cold winter months than in summer.

A widely used rule of thumb for raw meat is to start with 2 percent of the animal's weight and adjust from there. Whenever you're able to provide bones that are soft enough for the animal to chew through (lamb necks and shanks; chicken backs, wings, and drumsticks; chicken and turkey necks; oxtails; mutton ribs; and similar fare for dogs and poultry bones for cats), aim for 2.5 to 3 percent of the animal's weight. For a 50-pound dog, this would be 1 pound of raw meat, or 1¼ to 1½ pounds of raw meaty bones per day; for a 10-pound cat, this is 3 to 4 ounces of raw meat, or 4 to 5 ounces of raw meaty bones per day. Please note: If your pet is not used to raw bones, start with poultry neck bones, which are considered the "safest" bones. Dogs and cats with strong digestive tracts can eat just about anything, but most pets should be introduced to raw bones gradually.

Meat should be served to adult dogs and cats in large chunks or whole pieces, because this is how predators in the wild swallow meat. The only canines that eat something similar to ground meat are puppies who eat their parents' regurgitated stomach contents. Without large pieces of meat to keep them busy, stomach muscles atrophy and stomach secretions grow weak. Dogs and cats may need help digesting grains and vegetables, but they were designed to process chunks of raw meat and bone. More important, say the experts, without the exercise these foods provide, dogs are more likely to suffer from incomplete digestion, bloat, chronic diarrhea and other digestive disorders, as described on page 25.

What About Bones?

Dog owners often give bones to teething puppies and to older dogs as chew toys, but these bones are sterilized and far too large and hard to swallow. For complete nutrition, dogs and cats need bones they can chew through, swallow, and digest, just as their canine and feline cousins do in the wild.

Cooked bones are dangerous because they splinter and can cause serious problems. Raw bones are a different story. We're so indoctrinated by the "don't feed bones" rule that we forget dogs and cats have dined on them for thousands of years. Bones provide essential nutrients, hence the importance of bone meal as a pet food ingredient. But there's a world of difference between commercially processed bone meal and the raw bones your dog or cat might gnaw on.

When I switched my cats from cooked to raw food ten years ago, I had the same misgivings as anyone else, but Anitra Frazier's book *The Natural Cat*, my first guide, calmly recommended giving cats whole Rock Cornish game hens. I did and they loved them, bones and all. Pepper, Pumpkin II, and Samantha regularly share free-range chickens, and our only problem has been finding poultry shears strong enough to cut them into practical servings.

Holistic veterinarians warn that pets who are not used to eating bones or who are in poor health should start with small quantities. Too much at first may cause constipation, diarrhea, or digestion problems. In rare cases, poultry bones may violate the general rule that raw bones don't splinter, possibly because they are from older animals or because of their growing conditions. Necks provide the safest poultry bones for pets making the transition from commercial to raw foods.

After adjusting to an improved diet of fresh, raw foods, most dogs and cats are able to digest raw bones without difficulty. If bones are fed last, the rest of the meal acts as a cushion in the stomach.

Owners of medium-to-large dogs share a common first-time scenario. They tentatively offer a raw chicken neck or wing and watch helplessly as the excited dog leaps up and swallows it whole. Then they spend a sleepless night waiting for something terrible to happen. "My Golden Retrievers were so enthusiastic about raw bones," says trainer Nancy Strouss, "that I had to teach them how to chew. I did this by holding a chicken wing so tightly at one end that they had to gnaw on the other. After a few tries, they learned to chew through bones and not swallow them whole. In fact, I made it a command. Before giving a dog a bone, I say, 'Chew!' Now they know what it means."

In addition to their nutritional benefits, the gristle and tendons attached to raw bones are a natural dental floss, and crunching through raw bones is good for the teeth and gums. As veterinarian Beverly Cappel says, "You can always tell a bone-chewing dog; they have the whitest, strongest, cleanest teeth." Dogs and cats who eat raw, meaty bones save their owners the expense of tooth cleaning and other dental work; they rarely develop gum disease, and their breath is usually sweeter than that of their commercially fed relatives.

Even when they appreciate the benefits of raw bones, some owners are reluctant to provide them for personal reasons (bones can be messy and inconvenient) or because they have been frightened by veterinarians and other authority figures. Unfortunately, not feeding raw bones to dogs and cats may create nutritional imbalances that cause serious harm. In his book *Feed Your Pups with Bones*, Ian Billinghurst warns against the use of substitutes such as heat-sterilized bone meal and calcium supplements, for they can disrupt the natural balance of minerals in growing bodies and cause, instead of preventing, hip and elbow dysplasia and other structural problems.

There are more than a hundred important elements in raw bones, bone marrow, and connective tissue, all of which are vital to the health of joint cartilage, intervertebral discs, vascular walls, and other parts of the canine and feline body. Raw bones that are soft enough for your pet to bite through, swallow, and digest contain all of these nutrients, and a small number of commercial supplements made from cold-sterilized raw bones, including Wysong's Contifin and the Standard Process products Calcifood, Ostagen, and Biodent, contain most of them. If you are reluctant to feed your dog raw bones but want their nourishment, you can substitute either company's products (see Resources at the back of this book), or you can grind raw meaty bones in a meat grinder, which some breeders do as part of their puppies' first solid food. Keep in mind though, that supplements and freshly ground bones cannot provide the tooth-cleaning benefits, hours of chewing pleasure, or stomach exercise that raw meaty bones provide.

But I heard about a dog that . . . It's true. Animals *have* died from eating raw bones. After gorging themselves, some dogs have needed emergency surgery, prompting veterinarians to issue warnings. Others have needed veterinary care for problems caused by an accumulation of small, undigested pieces of bone in the stomach or intestines, and still others have died of acute gastric dilation, or bloat. Choking has occurred when raw bones got stuck in animals' throats.

In the April 1996 *Canine Journal*, an Australian publication, veterinary surgeon Tom Lonsdale wrote that when he was the veterinarian-in-attendance at a safari park, one of the lions under his care died suddenly. The cause of death was perforation of the intestine by a sharp section of ox vertebra. When a tigress fell ill, exploratory surgery showed raw bones impacting her bowel. Both animals were on a raw-meat diet, but the bones they swallowed had been cut with a saw, creating unnaturally sharp points and edges.

Even though the safari park staff agreed that raw meat and bones were the best foods for large carnivores despite the risks, Lonsdale became an advocate of canned food for domestic cats and dogs. In addition to being endorsed by veterinary organizations, these foods were safe. Nothing in them could perforate intestines, break teeth, or cause choking.

When members of what he calls the Raw Meaty Bone Lobby of concerned veterinarians called his attention to the link between his patients' poor health and their unnatural diet, Lonsdale stopped recommending canned food and began prescribing abundant fresh water, raw meaty bones, chicken wings, whole fish, and rabbit with small amounts of raw and cooked table scraps (minus any cooked bones) for both dogs and cats. Puppies and kittens received the same food mashed or grated in smaller, more frequent meals.

"Kittens and puppies begun early on a natural diet learn how to tackle their food and in our experience seldom require veterinary attention," he wrote in *Canine Journal*. Size is an important regulator of chewing function, for pieces cut too small permit the bone to be swallowed whole, risking obstruction, and large bones without meat provide less nutrition while increasing the risk of tooth wear and breakage.

Lonsdale and his colleagues noticed that many Australian pets that seemed to be suffering from old age had in fact developed an AIDS-like syndrome. "Happily, we found that the patients could be greatly improved by a change of diet," he wrote. In the December 1995 *British Journal of Small Animal Practice*, Lonsdale and his colleagues described this disorder and its successful treatment. "The animals were fed a raw meaty bone diet with occasional supplemental table scraps," the article explained. "The small dogs and cats received chicken wings, rabbit legs, and whole raw fish, whilst the larger dogs received lamb brisket, kangaroo tails, etc." All of the patients showed a speedy return to good health on this simple therapy.

One way to prevent problems in dogs or cats unfamiliar with raw bones is to teach them how to chew, as Nancy Strouss did with her Golden Retrievers. Bones that an animal can bite through are safer than those that are cut with a saw. Bones that are too large to swallow whole are safer than those that can be swallowed, although the size a dog might swallow whole decreases as she learns how to take her time and chew. Bones from young animals are less brittle than those from older animals, poultry neck bones are the least likely to cause problems, and serving bones after other foods provides a cushion that helps protect the stomach lining.

Supplementing an older pet or one that has been fed commercial food all his life with products containing hydrochloric acid (HCl) as well as animal-source digestive enzymes may help him digest raw bones. Keeping bones out of the reach of dogs that are literally starved for them prevents accidental overindulgences.

Other complaints about bones   Some owners complain that raw bones are messy. They're right. Samantha eats her bones on the kitchen floor or in her kennel, both of which are easy to clean. Some cats are so enthusiastic about raw meat that their owners feed them in the bathtub to keep things tidy. Although Pepper sometimes carries her dinner into the dining room, when fed separately she and Pumpkin II confine most of their stains to their placemats.

Occasionally, cats and dogs get bones stuck in their mouths, just as stick-chasing dogs sometimes lodge a twig or piece of wood between their teeth. In the September 1995 *Tiger Tribe*, an excellent magazine that is no longer published, Leslie Moran advised supervising the bone-feeding portion of the meal, especially if raw bones set off primal reactions such as aggressive or possessive behavior, growling, dragging the prize to a "safer" location, trying to steal another pet's food, or "creating a ferocious, savage mess while eating their bones." One of her cats wedged a piece of bone between the roof of his mouth and his lower jaw; another had difficulty separating the meat from a joint end and the long string of ligament attached to the bone made it impossible for him to chew or swallow. Both cats calmly resumed eating when she intervened. Had she not been present, the cats would no doubt have clawed these pieces free, just as their wild relatives do. A declawed cat is at an obvious disadvantage in such situations, in which case human supervision is an excellent idea.

Common sense makes all the difference in feeding raw bones to dogs and cats. As Moran wrote, feeding raw bones not only improves a pet's health, it is an important ritual linking animals through their genetic memory to a wild past.

But My Veterinarian Says . . .

Very few veterinarians recommend raw food or, for that matter, any home-prepared diet for dogs or cats. "That's because they don't know anything about nutrition," says Kathy Herman, who has bred four generations of Labrador Retrievers on raw food. "They go to vet schools that receive major funding from commercial pet food companies, the few nutrition classes they take are devoted to commercial pet foods, all their patients are on commercial pet foods, the only feeding trials they've conducted or read about used commercial food, and they simply don't know anything else. Home-prepared diets and raw foods frighten them because they're unfamiliar."

Lisa Freeman, D.V.M., Ph.D., a veterinary clinical nutritionist at Tufts University, finds much to criticize in home-prepared diets, and her views are widely shared. In the December 1998 *AKC Gazette*, the monthly magazine of the American Kennel Club, she wrote, "Although there are a variety of reasons why dog owners feed homemade diets, I generally try to steer owners away from them."

What's wrong with a home-prepared diet? Among other things, she wrote, "Many dogs have been spoiled by being fed treats or human food and now refuse dog food completely." Conventional veterinarians dislike variety, preferring to feed the same food at every meal every day. By this standard, practically every food, whether home-prepared or commercial, is nutritionally unbalanced. Instead of recommending variety, Freeman suggests having someone trained in canine nutrition evaluate a recipe to be sure it is nutritionally complete and then follow that recipe exactly. To owners concerned that their dogs will become bored with the same food day after day, she says, "With so many good foods on the market nowadays, an owner may change diets every few months or every year."

Even worse than home-cooked food, Freeman warns, is food that isn't cooked at all. "Some people recommend . . . raw meat diets for dogs," she wrote. "These are definitely not safe and you should not risk your dog's health by feeding them!"

Because America's veterinary schools emphasize the diagnosis of illness rather than the recognition of health, the suppression of symptoms rather than the prevention of disease, the routine use of commercial pet foods, and the same lack of nutritional education that affects our medical schools, it is not surprising that veterinary clinical nutritionists have such narrow views. Fresh, raw foods are not part of the veterinary culture, and veterinary authorities, like authorities in every field, reflect their cultural conditioning.

Celeste Yarnall, author of the books *Cat Care, Naturally* and *Natural Dog Care*, feeds her Tonkinese and Oriental Shorthair cats an all-raw diet and requires her kitten buyers to do the same. When one of her cats fell from a rooftop, his owner rushed him to an emergency clinic, where the veterinary staff marveled over his strong bones and excellent health. In fact, an attending veterinary technician realized that she had never seen a truly healthy cat before, and the following day she telephoned Yarnall to discuss her unusual (by veterinary standards) approach to feline health.

"The problem with veterinarians today," Yarnall told me, "is that the only animals they see eat nutritionally deficient food and get vaccinated every year. To them, a dog or cat that isn't dying of cancer is healthy, even though it may have eye and ear infections, skin and coat problems, allergies, poor muscle tone, structural defects, terrible teeth and gums, behavioral problems, and arthritis. These conditions are so common they're considered normal. Twenty-year-old cats are unusual today, and among pedigreed cats they are practically unheard of. In fact, it's getting hard to find cats who live to be nine or ten. I believe most feline and canine health problems stem from poor diet and overvaccination, and these are conditions an owner can control. While natural diet and holistic therapies can't cure everything, they can improve or prevent most common health disorders and help the animal live to an active old age.

"The only sensible strategy to follow," she concluded, "is to provide the food our pets were designed to consume. For dogs and cats, that means a constantly changing assortment of raw foods, especially raw meat. Veterinarians and pet food manufacturers are not the final authority on pet nutrition. Mother Nature is."

Preparing Raw Meat and Bones

Healthy dogs and cats in the wild can eat just about any raw meat and survive, if not thrive. Just think of all the bones dogs bury and all the birds and rodents cats consume. Their stomachs contain high concentrations of hydrochloric acid and digestive juices, and their digestive tracts host an abundance of beneficial bacteria, making it difficult for harmful bacteria to survive. Any meat, poultry, fish, or other fresh food that's suitable for human consumption should be safe for your dog or cat.

The following disinfecting methods are more for the protection of people than of pets, although any animal that's been fed only packaged, processed food may need protection from unfamiliar microbes until its digestive system recovers. Gum mastic, a Greek tree resin used for thousands of years as a digestive aid, has been shown to kill *E. coli, Salmonella,* and other harmful bacteria. Small amounts of gum mastic (½ gram per 50 pounds of body weight) or mastic essential oil (1 drop per 50 pounds) can be added to food or given with meals to dogs making the transition to a raw diet.

There are four ways to disinfect raw meat, raw bones, or eggs in the shell, listed below. The meat should be in large pieces and not ground. Keep meat and other perishable foods refrigerated until ready to use.

1. Soak the meat in a solution of ½ teaspoon original formula Clorox bleach per gallon of water for 15 to 20 minutes, then soak in plain water for 10 minutes.

2. Soak the meat in a sink or bowl containing cold water and several drops of 35 percent food-grade hydrogen peroxide. Use enough to create small bubbles in the water but not enough to change the meat's color. Soak for 10 minutes, then rinse in plain water.

3. Soak the meat in a sink or bowl containing cold water and 30 or more drops of liquid grapefruit seed extract; let stand 5 minutes and drain. Alternatively, add 20 or more drops to a 32-ounce spray bottle of filtered or distilled water, then spray on meat or poultry and rinse in clean water.

Any of the above methods also can be used to disinfect raw fruits and vegetables. Use a separate soak solution for each type of food.

4. Dip the meat in very hot water. In 1992, the *Journal of Epidemiology and Infection* reported that meat can be sterilized by placing it for 10 to 20 seconds in water that has been heated to 80 degrees C (176 degrees F). Doing so leaves the surface of the meat "virtually sterile." In a large pan, heat water just until active bubbles form at the bottom, or check the temperature with a kitchen thermometer; water at sea level reaches a rolling boil at 212 degrees F. Remove from heat. Holding the meat with tongs, immerse it for 10 to 20 seconds in the almost-boiling water. Let it drain in your pet's bowl.

At about 150 degrees F, hot water from the tap won't disinfect raw meat, but it will warm refrigerated meat to body temperature, a recommended step in meal preparation.

Soap and hot water effectively removes and destroys viruses, bacteria, and other harmful microbes from kitchen counters, floors, food bowls, cutting boards, utensils, refrigerator handles, and other surfaces. For information on natural disinfectants and their use, see pages 177 and 187.

Organ Meats

Organs are an important part of any carnivore's diet. In the wild, canines and felines consume most or all of the glands and organs of any animal they capture. Pet nutritionists agree that organ meats should make up a small, regular portion of the diet of both dogs and cats.

Liver is such a concentrated source of nutrients that it is often recommended for malnourished or ailing pets. As Donald R. Collins, D.V.M., wrote in the April 1993 *Natural Pet*, liver is sometimes called a mystery food or miracle food for its ability to save lives and improve health. A tablespoon of chopped liver added to their mothers' diet has saved many newborn puppies dying of "fading puppy syndrome." Orphan puppies stunted by inadequate infant formulas suddenly grow and gain weight when pureed liver is added to their food. Injured pets fed raw liver heal quickly, animals with a variety of serious illnesses recover faster, and pets with dull coats regain their luster.

Collins wrote that veterinary nutritionists have long referred to unidentified liver fractions and their dramatic effects on animal health. Raw beef and chicken liver are rich in protein, amino acids, phosphorus, potassium, copper, vitamin A, and B-complex vitamins including folic acid, pantothenic acid, vitamin B6, and choline. Because the liver stores toxins, it is important to feed liver from organically raised poultry and cattle. Raw liver can be pureed with water or juice and fed to animals on a modified fast.

Freeze-dried liver has been a popular training treat and between-meal snack in canine circles for years. But too much liver can cause problems, according to experts whose warnings have appeared in dog magazines. It is a good idea to alternate freeze-dried liver treats with other food rewards, to feed fresh liver not more than once or twice per week, to feed it in small servings, and to feed different types of liver. For example, if you give your dog several beef liver treats on Monday and Tuesday, wait until Friday to add raw chicken liver to her dinner.

In the past, dogs were fed raw bones, table scraps, and the parts of animals that weren't consumed by humans, such as the lungs, kidneys, heart, stomach, and entrails. During hunting season, some dogs are well supplied with glands and organs of deer and other wild game. Meat markets in ethnic neighborhoods sell a variety of organs. However, only a few American supermarkets carry organ meats other than liver and tripe. Even sweetbreads, which used to be popular, are now uncommon in suburban markets. Only a few American pet owners are comfortable handling unfamiliar meats, and just as important, not every dog or cat finds them appetizing.

Liver and other organ meats are so rich that some dogs vomit after eating them. "Start small" is always good advice. Although ground meat is not recommended for dogs or cats, grinding or pureeing is one way to introduce organ meats. Glands and organs are important foods, but they should be fed in small quantities on a rotating schedule and not every day.

Plates, Dishes, and Food Storage Materials

Food plates and water bowls should be glass, ceramic, or stainless steel, not aluminum, plastic, or pottery, which might contain lead glaze. The use of plastic food bowls has been associated with the loss of pigmentation on a dog's nose, and plastic is often mentioned as a cause of feline acne, a condition in which blackhead-like eruptions form on a cat's chin. Replacing plastic bowls with glass, ceramic, or stainless steel has cured these conditions in some dogs and cats.

Food and water bowls should be kept clean and well rinsed to remove soap residues that can contribute to chronic health problems. Dishes washed in a dishwasher receive ample rinsing, but dishes washed in a sink may not. One good habit is to rinse your pet's water bowl before filling it. Another is to rinse her food bowl, fill it with hot water, add her dinner portion of raw meat, and let it warm to body temperature before draining. Both practices remove lingering soap residues and promote good digestion.

Ever since researchers discovered possible links between aluminum, Alzheimer's disease, and other debilitating illnesses, health-conscious consumers have questioned the use of aluminum cookware, foil, bowls, and utensils. Aluminum is the earth's most abundant metallic element, but it is so reactive that it does not naturally occur as a free metal. Almost any substance that comes in contact with aluminum, including air and water, will form aluminum compounds. These reactions are most likely to occur rapidly at high temperatures or in the presence of acids. Dogs and cats on an all-raw diet are not endangered by aluminum cookware, but aluminum water bowls, food bowls, storage containers, and foil may put them at risk. Raw meat and other foods wrapped in freezer paper before being sealed in aluminum foil are protected from this chemical reaction.

Plastic wrap, considered by many a safe alternative to aluminum foil, may be dangerous in a different way. In January 1999, the *New York Times* reported that plastic wrap used throughout the grocery industry contains a potentially harmful chemical, DEHA, that can leach into food, especially high-fat food, on contact. DEHA belongs to a family of chemicals shown to disrupt hormone balance in animals.

Ten years ago British manufacturers replaced DEHA with a safer plasticizer. Scientists at Consumers Union and the Natural Resources Defense Council recommend that American manufacturers do the same. Some have. In a separate test of seven national and store brands, Consumers Union found that only Reynolds Wrap was made with DEHA.

To reduce your family's (and your pet's) exposure to DEHA, food safety experts recommend that you remove cling wrap immediately from cheese or meat, then store it in a plastic bag or container. Thinly slice and discard the outer layer of hard cheese and scrape off a thin layer of meat— and don't give the scrapings to your pet. When purchasing meat from a butcher, ask that it be wrapped in paper. If using cling wrap to cover food in a ceramic bowl, make sure it doesn't touch the food.

Combating Bloat

Bloat is such a mysterious condition that it is impossible to predict which dogs will succumb to it and for what reason. Although its cause is unknown, researchers have linked it with the consumption of commercial foods, especially large meals of dry dog food. The condition usually develops in adult dogs two to six hours after eating, when the upper abdominal area becomes enlarged with gas and liquid, in some cases making the skin feel as tight as a drum. Symptoms include excessive salivation, drooling, frantic attempts to eat grass and vomit, extreme restlessness and discomfort, increasing weakness, dehydration, shock, and in some cases torsion, a severe twisting or rotation of the stomach that blocks its entry and exit.

Bloat can be prevented by feeding large chunks of raw meat, bones, and other hard foods that require the stomach to work. This provides regular exercise that strengthens the muscles and "massages" the stomach and bowels. Diane Laratta discovered this approach in 1984 when she met Connecticut veterinarian H. J. Van Kruiningen, D.V.M., Ph.D. In the preceding fifteen years, Laratta had bred seven consecutive litters of Standard Poodles and eleven of her dogs, including at least one from each litter, developed bloat. Most of them died.

In his lectures and veterinary journal papers, Van Kruiningen recommended feeding raw chicken, whole raw fruits, and raw vegetables three to four times per week as a bloat-prevention strategy. "I was highly motivated," Laratta told me, "but in those days I wasn't comfortable with raw chicken, so I gave them apples, carrots, and other hard vegetables."

After Laratta adopted this feeding plan, none of her Poodles developed bloat. "I made copies of Dr. Kruiningen's articles and gave them to everyone, especially people who were taking a puppy or adopting one of my older dogs," she said. "So far the only cases of bloat have occurred in dogs whose owners put them on a straight commercial diet with no fruits and vegetables. In one case, it happened within a month."

Although the stereotypical bloat victim is a large-breed dog who breaks into a bag of kibble when no one's looking, bloat can affect a wide range of breeds and sizes, including German Shepherd Dogs, Irish Setters, Great Danes, St. Bernards, Bloodhounds, Boxers, Weimaraners, Collies, Doberman Pinschers, and mixed-breed dogs of similar ancestry. Basset Hounds, Dachshunds, Standard Poodles, Golden Retrievers, Labrador Retrievers, and other breeds, although less susceptible, have also succumbed. The same disease can occur in cats, guinea pigs, rats, mice, and other animals, including humans. Van Kruiningen's research implicates mono-diets in which the same food is given every day at every meal, greedy eaters, large meals, commercially prepared foods containing refined cereal grains or soy beans, fermentive gastric flora, and abnormal gastric function as the primary causes of bloat.

Even if your dog isn't from one of the breeds associated with bloat, it's a good idea to make meals as relaxing as possible. In the February 1999 edition of her *Dog Love Letter*, veterinarian Beverly Cappel wrote that dogs are genetically programmed to compete for food to survive, causing them to eat fast, especially when under stress. An obvious source of stress is the presence of other animals, but it can also come from children playing or people coming and going, which produces a heightened state of alert in a dog whose job is to protect her extended family. "She can't protect her pack and eat at the same time," says Cappel, "so she quickly eats her food."

To slow a too-fast eater, Cappel suggests scheduling meals at quiet times in a relaxed atmosphere and distracting the dog every few bites by calling her name or giving her a special treat such as a small piece of cheese. "The goal is to make the eating less frantic and prevent her from swallowing air," she explains. "Have some patience and gradually she will learn to eat slowly and steadily."

The easiest way to slow a dog's eating is to give her foods too large to swallow without chewing, such as very large pieces of meat and raw meaty bones. As Cappel noted, one reason that wolves and other wild predators aren't prone to gastric bloat and torsion is that they have to chew their meat, which slows their eating.

In some cases, prescription drugs have caused bloat by preventing normal digestion. After one of Nancy Strouss's Golden Retrievers was given powerful antacids to treat an inflamed stomach lining, undigested meals accumulated in her stomach. Strouss recognized the panting dog's symptoms and rushed her to the veterinarian in time to save her life.

Occasionally, bloat occurs for no apparent reason. Sarah Wilson, who raises German Shepherd Dogs, has a friend in the breed who got up one morning, checked her dog as she walked past his kennel and returned half an hour later to find him dying of bloat. "No one can explain why," she told me. "It's tempting to dwell on whatever the dog ate last, but that may have nothing to do with it. Stress is an important factor in bloat and one that's often overlooked. Dogs are stressed by unexpected events, travel, changes in residence, and anything that disrupts their normal routines. I knew a Great Dane that died of bloat while staying with his show handler. Things like this are no one's fault, they just happen."

One technique Wilson developed while running a boarding kennel years ago is to percuss each dog after dinner by gently and firmly tapping it up one side and down the other until it burps. "Yes," she says laughing, "just like burping a baby. Bloat might or might not have anything to do with air trapped in the stomach. All I can say is that the dogs enjoyed it, and despite being under a great deal of stress, being on a diet of dry commercial pet food, and being from breeds prone to it, none of them ever developed bloat."

It may be possible to interrupt a developing case of bloat with the use of essential oils that are both safe for topical application and recommended for indigestion, such as chamomile, or a blend of lavender and peppermint. These oils need not be given orally; they can be applied to a dog's feet, neck, or abdomen, several drops at a time for rapid absorption into the bloodstream. Although essential oils may not be able to untwist a torsioned stomach, their fast-acting therapeutic benefits may relieve bloat before torsioning occurs. See page 178.

Drinking Water

The purity of your pet's drinking water is a serious consideration. Alfred Plechner, author of *Pet Allergies*, was one of the first to warn pet owners that contaminated drinking water is a common cause of health problems. As many holistic veterinarians have since reported, the simple act of replacing tap water with clean water has brought rapid, dramatic improvements to the health of many dogs and cats.

Some nutritionists swear by distilled water, while others condemn it for its lack of minerals. Some say that charcoal filters are all you need, and others say they're worse than useless. Everyone has something bad to say about plastic containers, but some spring water is sold in clear (not opaque or cloudy) plastic jugs, which are more stable and prevent the plastic taste that migrates into water from opaque bottles.

Whatever you can do to improve your pet's—and your own—water is worth the effort. If you use a charcoal filter on your kitchen faucet, change it more often than the instructions indicate. If you use a home distiller, it's probably a good idea to add colloidal minerals to help compensate for their lack. Health magazines often report on water safety and home treatment methods; look for these at newsstands or check your local library.

Once you have a good source of drinking water, consider adding small amounts of Willard Water concentrate (see pages 87 and 88) and a pinch of unrefined sea salt (see page 76) to improve it further.

Making Grain and Seeds Digestible

Although dogs and cats are not designed to eat cooked food, they are not designed to digest raw grain and seeds, either. Pet nutritionist Pat McKay says, "The only grain they can utilize has been predigested, the way it is in horse manure or regurgitated stomach contents—but I don't think America's pet owners are ready to provide either of these excellent sources of grain nutrition."

Fortunately, there is another way. Sprouting changes grain and seeds into living foods rich in vitamins, trace minerals, enzymes, amino acids, and other nutrients. Grinding or pureeing the sprouts makes them easier to digest, and so does adding raw honey (a natural source of amylase, an enzyme that digests carbohydrates) or an enzyme powder that contains amylase (health food stores and pet supply stores sell several brands). The sprouting process releases amylase from grain, but dogs and cats previously fed a commercial diet may need a little extra while their digestive systems make the transition to natural fare.

How to Sprout Grain

To sprout grain, buy organically raised wheat, rye, spelt, kamut, barley, oats, or buckwheat from a health food store, macrobiotic supply company, or sprout catalog.

Soak ½ to 1 cup grain in a wide-mouth quart canning jar of water to which you have added 5 or 6 drops of grapefruit seed extract. Soak wheat, buckwheat, oats, barley, sunflower seeds, and other large grains ten to twelve hours or overnight. Eight hours is recommended for medium seeds and about five hours for small seeds. For increased mineral content, add a pinch of powdered or liquid kelp, a splash of Willard Water concentrate (see page 87), or several drops of liquid trace minerals. Adding an ounce of 3 percent hydrogen peroxide is another technique for increasing germination.

Health food stores sell plastic sprouting lids for wide-mouth quart jars, or you can fashion a sprouting lid with cheesecloth and a rubber band or with a wire mesh strainer. With sprouting lid in place, drain the jar well, then lay it on its side in a warm place away from direct sunlight. Ideal sprouting temperatures are between 70 and 80 degrees F.

After twenty-four to forty-eight hours, you will see small white roots emerging from the grain. (If you don't see this growth on almost every seed by the second day, your grain is not viable and should be discarded.) Let it grow another day, then puree the grain in a blender or food processor. If desired, add a teaspoon to a tablespoon of raw honey (a source of carbohydrate-digesting amylase) and/or ¼ teaspoon of enzyme powder and let the mash stand at room temperature for an hour or two before refrigerating to better approximate the contents of a prey animal's stomach. For dogs, start with 1 teaspoon per 10 pounds of body weight every other day and gradually increase to twice this amount. For cats, start with ¼ teaspoon per 10 pounds of body weight every other day and gradually increase to twice this amount. Like other dietary recommendations, these are very general suggestions. Let common sense be your guide, increasing or decreasing the amounts suggested here as appropriate for your animal.

How to Sprout Seeds

Green sprouts, once exotic fare, are now mainstream. They're sold in supermarkets and are used to garnish salads and sandwiches in fast-food restaurants. At least one sprouting seed, the chia, is sold as a novelty; it grows like a fuzzy green fur over terra-cotta animals called Chia Pets.

Seed sprouts are easy to grow, and the green foliage they produce is an important source of vitamins, minerals, enzymes, and other nutrients. To sprout alfalfa, buckwheat, cabbage, chia, chive, clover, fenugreek, radish, sunflower, and other seeds, soak them overnight as described on page 30. Most seeds sold for sprouting are, in addition to being organically grown and untreated, tested for *Salmonella* and other contaminants. One easy way to prevent the growth of harmful bacteria is to add a drop or two of grapefruit seed extract to the jar before you add the seeds. Add just enough water to cover the seeds and stir well, then fill to the top with water. Soak the seeds for several hours or overnight and drain well.

If using glass jars for sprouting, set the jar on its side, with the plastic sprout lid or cheesecloth top in place. If using a sprouting tray system or fabric sprouting bag, follow the manufacturer's directions. If using a bamboo basket, rinse it well, empty the seeds into the basket, rinse again, drain well, and place the basket in a large plastic bag left partly open. This creates a greenhouse that allows air to circulate but prevents the seed from drying out. Your use of grapefruit seed extract in the soaking water should prevent mold, but if it occurs, rinse the seeds vigorously under a strong spray, drain well, then spray the sprouts with 3 percent hydrogen peroxide or diluted grapefruit seed extract.

Unlike sprouting grains, seeds need rinsing at least twice a day. Run cold water over the sprouts in a colander or fill the sprouting jar with cold water and shake it. Return the sprouts to their tray or jar as necessary.

If your sprouting area is dark, move the growing sprouts into indirect sunlight on the third or fourth day.

If growing a crop that produces empty hulls, such as alfalfa, radish, or red clover, wait until the hulls begin to separate and fall off, then submerge the sprouts in a sink of cool water and agitate them. Empty hulls will separate from the sprouts and either sink to the bottom or float to the surface. If using a bamboo basket, simply submerge and agitate the basket (the sprouts will cling by their roots) and let it drain; if using a jar, lift the sprouts into a strainer, then return them to the jar.

While just-sprouting legumes can be difficult to digest, fully sprouted peas and other legumes turn green and leafy, producing "pea lettuce," which can be chopped or pureed and added to your pet's food just like other green sprouts.

Buying Sprouts

If using purchased sprouts such as those sold in supermarkets, rinse them well under cold running water. Although rare, *Salmonella, E. coli,* and other harmful bacteria have been found in some commercial sprouts and salad ingredients. To guard against bacterial contamination, spray or soak sprouts in a dilute solution of grapefruit seed extract before rinsing.

Raw legume sprouts, including alfalfa, beans, peas, and clover, have received negative publicity in recent years because they contain toxins that are not destroyed during digestion. These include saponins, which are chemicals that can damage red blood cells, and canavanine, a toxin that can harm the immune system and possibly increase the risk of cancer and degenerative diseases. The toxic effects of canavanine are known as lathyrism, after the botanical genus of the sweet pea, *Lathyrus,* which contains a similar toxin. Lathyrism, which closely resembles systemic lupus erythematosus, or SLE, a serious autoimmune disorder, is a recognized illness in India, where it is seen in people who consume large quantities of chickpea (garbanzo bean) flour. When cooked, as for the Middle Eastern spread hummus, chickpeas are safe, but chickpea flour is made from beans that are dry-roasted, a process that does not destroy the toxin. Proponents of raw-food diets maintain that the complex nutrients in raw green sprouts prevent any single toxin from causing harm. More important, they note that the alfalfa used in the canavanine research was one- to three-day-old not-yet-green germinating seedlings that were oven-dried to reduce their bulk. According to sprouting authority Sam Graci in the July 1998 edition of *Alive* magazine, no tests were done with mature green alfalfa sprouts. "Recent research shows that L-canavanine (which is also present in onions, garlic, and soybean seeds) rapidly decreases in plants as they mature during germination," wrote Graci. "L-canavanine in a mature alfalfa sprout represents only a 0.00075 percent concentration. Don't doubt the sprout!"

Some researchers claim broccoli sprouts contain chemicals that reduce the risk of cancer and other serious illnesses. As a result of the increased demand for broccoli sprouts, they are appearing in supermarkets and health food stores, and broccoli seeds are now sold for sprouting.

For more information about sprout growing, see the Resources at the back of this book.

Fresh Wheat Grass and Other Cereal Grasses

Both cats and dogs are known to have a fondness for grass. Pumpkin, my husband's first red tabby, loved to sleep in trays of wheat grass growing under full-spectrum lights in our basement during snowy winters. Pet supply stores sell kits for growing oat, wheat, and rye grass for cats. Dogs are so known for their grass cravings that one wild grass is called dog grass in their honor. Yes, some dogs eat grass in an effort to throw up, but that isn't its only purpose. In addition to mincing the grass you add to their dinners, give your pets an occasional handful of green grass or let them harvest it themselves.

Once a soaked grain begins to sprout, you can plant it in potting soil in a plastic planting tray, restaurant tray, lined cardboard box, flowerpot, or any container between 1 and 2 inches deep with no drainage holes. Fill trays with an inch of potting soil or garden compost; fill flowerpots to the top.

Water the planting tray's soil until moist but not wet. Spread the seeds in a thin layer, over the entire surface. Cover with an inverted tray or with a wet paper towel covered with plastic to keep light out and moisture in. After two days, remove the cover, water the sprouting greens, and place them outside in indirect light for another two days, then move them into direct sunlight. In cold weather, place trays under full-spectrum plant lights indoors. Water daily until the grass is about 6 inches high, which takes about a week. If mold forms on the soil's surface from overwatering, spray the grass with 3 percent hydrogen peroxide or with 1 part liquid grapefruit seed extract diluted in 4 to 6 parts water.

Harvest grass by cutting it with scissors or a knife just above the soil surface. It will keep well in the refrigerator for about a week in self-sealing bags that you press the air out of or wrapped in layers of damp newspapers or paper towels. After harvesting, recycle the soil mat by placing it in your compost bin and start over.

For more about cereal grasses, see page 81.

Dairy Products

Raw milk, especially raw goat's milk, is one of the most widely prescribed foods for puppies, kittens, cats, and dogs. If you have access to organically produced raw milk, cheese, or butter, you may want to provide this food. Do not feed your pet pasteurized, homogenized, condensed, septic-packaged, "long life," or sweetened condensed milk, all of which have been shown to cause health problems in dogs and cats. By eliminating dairy products, many pet owners have prevented common allergies and ear infections. No adult animal in the wild has a reliable source of milk, and after weaning, dogs and cats lose their ability to produce lactase, the enzyme that digests lactose, or milk sugar. The symptoms of a lactose intolerance include bloating, gas, flatulence, diarrhea, and abdominal discomfort.

Yogurt, kefir, and other fermented milk products are often recommended for dogs and cats because they contain beneficial bacteria, but unless they are freshly made, these products contain few viable bacteria.

Your pet will derive more benefits from acidophilus and other probiotic supplements as well as from the foods that feed them (see below), especially if he has been treated with antibiotics.

Fresh Herbs and Vegetables

Parsley, sage, thyme, rosemary, oregano, purslane, cleavers, comfrey, dandelion greens, collard greens, wheat grass, buckwheat grass, and other green herbs are appropriate for both dogs and cats, but unlike humans and vegetation-eating animals, dogs and cats cannot digest cellulose. Whole raw vegetables pass through their bodies almost unchanged. An intermediate step is necessary to help break down cellulose cells.

Puree, finely grind, or grate vegetables or put them through a juicer. Some markets and health food stores sell frozen, organically grown carrot juice; many health food stores have juice bars equipped with macerating juicers or hydraulic juice presses, which produce juice that keeps for several days without losing nutrients; or you can make your own at home. If you use a centrifugal or macerating juicer, save the pulp for your pet. Because leftover pulp does not keep well, try to use it within a few hours, or freeze it in ice cube trays, transferring the frozen cubes to a plastic freezer bag for long-term storage.

You also can slice, grate, chop, or puree cucumbers, carrots, or other vegetables, layer them with a small amount of unrefined sea salt, and press them under a weight, such as a heavy plate. This creates lactic acid fermentation, which improves digestion, increases the absorption of nutrients, feeds the beneficial bacteria that live in your pet's intestines, and may reduce the risk of cancer, bowel disease, and other illnesses. Let the vegetables stand until their juice separates out as a clear liquid that covers them and the vegetables develop a piquant flavor. Add small amounts of the clear juice to your pet's drinking water, and puree or blend the vegetables before adding them to your pet's dinner. "Whichever way you do it," says Ian Billinghurst, in his book *Give Your Dog a Bone*, "the end result is a raw food, a vegetable pulp that your pet easily digests for brilliant, healthy nutrition."

How large should the vegetable servings be? Pat McKay, Celeste Yarnall, Anitra Frazier, and many other pet nutritionists recommend vegetables as 20 to 30 percent of the total daily food allowance for a dog or cat. Kymythy Schultze, who worked as a wildlife rehabilitator and who uses wild prey as the model for her raw feeding plan, recommends much smaller amounts.

"The main source of vegetable matter for wild canines and felines is the contents of their prey's stomachs," she explains, "and if you take a close look at prey animals, their stomachs are not very large. I find that when we start giving our dogs and cats too much vegetable matter, we can make their system over-alkaline, which can lead to problems. Most of a prey animal's body consists of muscle meat and bones, with a few small organs and whatever food is in the digestive tract. I encourage my students to follow the proportions of their species' typical prey animals, such as rabbits for dogs and mice for cats, and to avoid feeding large servings of fruit and vegetables."

Convenience Foods and Emergency Rations

What if you're in a hurry, or didn't have time to stop at the store? What if your husband/wife/parents/friends/neighbors/children insist on giving Fido or Fluffy a dog biscuit, cat treat, or other not-raw, not-at-all-natural tidbit?

Relax. A few deviations here and there won't derail your feeding plan. Pepper, Pumpkin II, and Samantha have had their share of all-meat baby food and other emergency rations. The next day we're back on track. I think of minced wheat grass, garlic, and enzyme powders as antidotes to processed convenience foods.

If you have to choose between a frozen or cooked food, or between a microwaved or boiled food, which is better? Foods can be warmed to a few degrees above body temperature without damaging heat-sensitive vitamins, trace minerals, enzymes, amino acids, and other "fresh factors," but the temperatures required for pasteurization (131 to 158 degrees F) or reached in baking, boiling, frying, poaching, canning, and high-temperature drying have deleterious effects.

Fresh is almost always best, but when that's not possible, keep this list in mind. From best to worst:

- Fresh, served raw (most desirable).
- Frozen and thawed, served raw.
- Freeze-dried or dried at low temperature.
- Lightly steamed or scalded, not heated through.
- Fried, baked, boiled, pasteurized, or dried at high temperatures.
- Microwaved, irradiated, pressure-cooked, or canned under pressure (least desirable).

You can create your own convenience dinners by preparing more than one meal at a time and refrigerating single servings in self-sealing plastic bags, glass bowls, or other containers. Gently warm refrigerated food by placing it in hot water, placing its serving bowl in hot water, or gently heating the food in a double boiler until it's somewhere between room and body temperature.

In the 1930s, the French chemist Paul Kouchakoff discovered that as soon as cooked or processed food is tasted, white blood cells rush to the intestines. This phenomenon, called digestive leucocytosis, disrupts the immune system; the body regards cooked food as a pathogen and works hard to destroy it. When Kouchakoff's volunteers ate raw food, their white blood cells remained in place. As Leslie and Susannah Kenton write in *Raw Energy*, every time white blood cells flock to the intestines to deal with cooked food, the rest of the body is left undefended. "Continual red alerts, three or more times a day, year in and year out," they observe, "put considerable strain on the immune system."

If you eat something cooked after eating something raw, however, leucocytosis doesn't happen. The body responds only to the first bite of food. For that reason, it's sensible to begin every meal with a taste of something raw. If you have to feed your pet something that has been pasteurized, baked, canned, boiled, or heated above body temperature, give her a raw food first, such as a carrot or even a piece of grass to nibble on. In addition, to help compensate for the lack of fresh factors in food that has been heated, add an enzyme powder.

Menu Planning

The notion that every meal an animal eats should be completely balanced came into vogue with the use of packaged foods. If you were restricted to the same food in the same amount every day for the rest of your life, each identical meal would have to be nutritionally balanced because you would have no other source of nutrients. But you don't eat that way, you don't feed your children that way, and animals in the wild don't eat that way, either. It's completely unnatural. What matters is not whether tonight's dinner contains 100 percent of every nutrient your body requires but whether all of the combined foods you eat today or this week provide them.

Monotony is not only boring, it's dangerous. Cats who eat only tuna and dogs who eat only one kind of meat eventually suffer serious health problems. So do pets who eat the same processed food at every meal.

The chemical analysis of commercial pet food ingredients is meaningless no matter what their origin because commercial pet foods are cooked, and, as Francis Pottenger proved more than sixty years ago, cooked food is deficient by definition. A variety of high-quality meats, bones, and other foods served raw or minimally processed in combination with a minimum of nutritional supplements supplies everything a dog or cat needs for perfect health. Why feed your pet under laboratory-controlled conditions when its species evolved on a constantly changing assortment of foods? Yes, cats require more protein than dogs, but neither needs a computer-equipped lab technician for basic menu planning.

The first American veterinarian to write a best-selling book on holistic pet care was Richard Pitcairn, D.V.M., whose *Natural Health for Dogs and Cats* was published in 1982. Although he recommended feeding raw meat, raw bones, and other raw fare, Pitcairn's recipes included ample quantities of cooked grains, cooked beans, and cooked potatoes, and several recommended cooking, steaming, or baking eggs, meat, and fish. In fact, most of the recipes would have looked at home in a cookbook for humans.

Pitcairn was not alone in recommending ingredients and preparation techniques familiar to his readers and clients. Anitra Frazier's 1983 book, *The Natural Cat*, discussed food at length and recommended feeding 60 percent raw ground beef or cooked meat, 20 percent steamed or grated vegetables, and 20 percent cooked grain, plus vitamin, mineral, and enzyme supplements. Most of the holistic pet care books and magazine articles that followed used similar proportions and ingredients. In the early 1980s, when few Americans had any idea what *holistic* meant, an all-raw diet based on meat and bones was, for most pet owners, far more radical than it seems today.

The contrast between the complicated dishes recommended for pets fifteen years ago and the streamlined approach of today's leading pet nutritionists is startling. In her 1998 book *The Ultimate Diet*, Kymythy Schultze combines raw meat, raw bones, a small amount of raw pureed vegetables, and tiny amounts of "extras" such as cod liver oil, kelp, alfalfa, vitamin C, and occasional organ meats. No dairy products, grains, legumes, nuts, or fruits appear in her basic recipes, although fruits and nuts can be used as optional ingredients or occasional treats. There are no complicated schedules of nutritional supplements because, as Schultze's nutritional tables show, this diet is rich in the nutrients dogs and cats require for optimum health. The diet advocated by Ian Billinghurst and like-minded veterinarians is almost identical, consisting of raw meaty bones, occasional raw eggs or ripe fruits, small amounts of pureed vegetables, and other extras such as kelp, brewer's yeast, herbs, and table scraps.

While writing *The Encyclopedia of Natural Pet Care,* I interviewed several veterinarians who were concerned about the nutritional balance of raw-meat diets because of patients who developed serious health problems, vitamin deficiencies, and mineral imbalances on such fare. Most or all of these dogs and cats, however, ate a single type of meat, usually ground beef, in combination with cooked grains, and none of them ate raw bones.

Providing a well-balanced, species-appropriate, natural raw diet does not involve complicated ingredient lists or hours of preparation. In fact, as Pat McKay is fond of saying, "If it takes more than ten minutes a day, you either love to be in the kitchen or you're doing something wrong."

Feeding the Adult Dog

The following are guidelines for adult dogs of most breeds. Feed one or two meals per day and nothing between meals. Depending on your dog's training schedule, the latter instruction may be unrealistic, but the fewer between-meal snacks, the better. Supplements can be given with either meal. If your dog is exceptionally active, like working Retrievers during hunting season, feed as much and as often as necessary.

Quantities depend on many factors: breed, size, metabolism, exercise and workload, even the weather. Working Alaskan sled dogs need thousands of calories a day, while warm-weather couch potatoes need hardly any. Large dogs need more, small dogs less. Dogs fed a natural diet are guided by an internal appetite control that directs them to eat as much as they need and then stop, so once your dog is used to fresh, raw food, your best guide will be his appetite. A general rule of thumb is to feed a daily ration of 2 to 3 percent of the dog's body weight in bones and meat. For a 50-pound dog, this would be about 1 to 1½ pounds of bones and meat. Start with approximately this amount and adjust as needed.

A week of menus for a 50-pound dog. Serve any of the following to a dog who spends an hour or more in active outdoor exercise. Increase the quantity and/or selection for more active or larger dogs; decrease for less

BREAKFAST OR MIDDAY SNACK

Monday:	1 banana.
Tuesday:	1 avocado sprinkled with unrefined sea salt.
Wednesday:	¼ cup sprouting grain blended or pureed with ½ cup raw milk or juice.
Thursday:	½ cup raw-milk cheese.
Friday:	1 raw egg, including shell.
Saturday:	1 apple or mango.

DINNER

Cut meat into large chunks if necessary; otherwise, simply give your dog a whole turkey thigh, chicken back, and so forth. Warm food as described on page 37.

Monday:	1 pound raw beef (not ground). 2 tablespoons herbal puree (see page 132). 1 teaspoon cod liver oil. 1 teaspoon kelp blend (see page 93).
Tuesday:	1½ pounds raw lamb neck bones. 1 tablespoon sprouted grain blend (see page 93).
Wednesday:	1 pound raw chicken breast, wings, neck, or legs, bones and all, plus the chicken's liver and heart. 4 tablespoons carrot juice or pressed grated carrots (see page 35).
Thursday:	1 pound raw fish or fish that has been lightly steamed or baked (add an enzyme powder if the fish isn't raw). 1 teaspoon cod liver oil. ¼ cup pureed pressed vegetables.
Friday:	1¼ pounds raw turkey thighs, wings, or drumsticks, including bones. 1 teaspoon kelp blend.
Saturday:	1¼ pounds raw beef ribs or oxtails (bones and meat). 2 minced garlic cloves. ¼ cup pureed pressed vegetables.

active or smaller dogs. Serve different foods for breakfast every day to ensure variety. Supply clean, pure water throughout the day. Please remember that these menus are offered only as examples, not as a regimented feeding plan. Substitute whatever ingredients are on sale or readily available. Whenever possible, ingredients should be organically raised. No menu is listed for Sunday, which is a water-only fast day. (Young puppies, very small breeds, and dogs with a very fast metabolism should not be fasted for more than half a day; consult a holistic veterinarian before fasting any dog that has a serious illness.)

Breakfast is an optional meal, for healthy adult dogs can eat a single meal per day. The foods listed for breakfast can be given at any time of day as an occasional treat. (See sidebar on page 41.)

The following are optional ingredients: herbal powders as appropriate, enzyme supplements, glandular supplements, trace minerals, unrefined sea salt, vitamin and/or mineral supplements, acidophilus supplements, and other products described in chapter 2, as well as herbal preparations described in chapter 3.

Feeding Puppies

Feed puppies and small dogs the same basic foods, but in smaller portions and cut into smaller pieces. Give them bones that are easy for them to chew through, such as chicken necks. Teething puppies enjoy gnawing on chicken wings and, if available, raw carob pods. Very young puppies can be fed three or four times per day; by six months, puppies can be fed twice per day. Ian Billinghurst and other veterinarians warn against overfeeding, for although a fat, glossy pup may look adorable, a leaner, hungry puppy is more likely to avoid common growth and health problems.

Please see my *Encyclopedia of Natural Pet Care* for the feeding of pregnant or lactating bitches and infant puppies.

Feeding the Adult Cat

Like healthy dogs, healthy adult cats can eat a single meal per day. To stimulate your cat's digestive organs, pet nutritionists recommend engaging in the same pre-meal activity every day, such as playing with toys that bring out your cat's prey-hunting instincts. At our house, brushing is part of the dinnertime ritual.

A week of menus for a 10-pound house cat. Adjust the following quantities as needed for larger, smaller, younger, older, and less or more

Monday: ¼ pound raw chicken or game hen with bones (include the liver and/or other organs if available). Pinch of powdered seaweed (kelp, dulse, etc.). ½ teaspoon cod liver oil.

Tuesday: ¼ pound raw beef or lamb cut into large chunks. 1 teaspoon to 1 tablespoon finely minced or pureed fresh wheat grass, dandelion, or other greens. 1 teaspoon flaxseed oil. Pinch of unrefined sea salt.

Wednesday: ¼ pound raw or lightly steamed fish. ⅛ teaspoon enzyme supplement powder. 1 teaspoon pureed sprouted grain (see page 30.) ½ teaspoon cod liver oil. Pinch of unrefined sea salt.

Thursday: ¼ pound raw chicken with bones. 1 or 2 ounces raw goat's milk or raw-milk cheese if available. Pinch of unrefined sea salt. 1 teaspoon herbal puree (see page 132). ½ teaspoon flaxseed oil.

Friday: ¼ cup raw or lightly steamed fish plus 1 raw egg. Pinch of unrefined sea salt. 1 teaspoon pureed sprouted grain. ½ teaspoon cod liver oil.

Saturday: ¼ pound raw turkey cut into large chunks. Include the turkey neck if available. 1 teaspoon finely minced or pureed wheat grass or other herbs. 1 teaspoon cod liver oil.

active cats. Combine ingredients and warm the food slightly before serving. Try to feed something different every day so that your cat consumes a variety of foods. If you decide to feed two meals per day, divide the day's allotment of food into two servings and give half in the morning and half at night.

When cut into pieces for serving, 1 ounce by weight is approximately 2 or 3 rounded tablespoons; 4 ounces by weight is a little more than ⅔ cup. It is not necessary to measure ingredients with precision because the goal is to emulate Mother Nature, and animals in the wild never consume the same foods in the same amounts at every meal.

Let your cat determine how much food to supply. Give as much as the animal will eat in fifteen to twenty minutes, then remove the food. Supply only water between meals.

The following are optional ingredients: 1 minced garlic clove or capsule equivalent, herbal powders as appropriate, enzyme supplements, glandular supplements, trace mineral supplements, vitamin and/or mineral supplements, acidophilus supplements, and other supplements described in chapter 2, as well as herbal preparations described in chapter 3.

Occasionally offer raw watermelon, cantaloupe, cucumber, mango, banana, avocado, or other ripe raw fruit. Some cats love raw corn, which should be pureed and mixed with an enzyme powder containing amylase for improved digestion. Encourage your cat to eat a variety of fresh, raw foods, no matter how unlikely they may seem.

Feeding Kittens

Feed very young kittens three or four times per day using the same basic meals served in tiny pieces and small servings. If raw goat's milk is available, give it in place of meat once or twice per day if desired.

By the age of six months, healthy kittens can be fed twice per day. Avoid overfeeding kittens; kittens should be lean rather than fat and slightly hungry rather than sated.

Please see my *Encyclopedia of Natural Pet Care* for information regarding the feeding of pregnant or lactating cats and infant kittens.

Forget It! My Fluffy Won't Eat That!

Sure she will. She just needs time to get used to the change. Help her by introducing new foods slowly in tiny quantities, adding them to what she already eats.

Many owners make the transition from commercial to raw foods so gradually that it takes weeks or months. Others, like Cathy Winkler, do it literally overnight. "I used to feed my Portuguese Water Dogs kibble with all kinds of supplements," she told me, "but I wasn't happy with that, so one day I just quit. My dogs, which ranged in age from puppies to nine years old, were basically healthy and we went cold turkey. One day they were eating dry food out of a bag and the next they were eating raw meat and raw bones. They thought they'd died and gone to heaven, and we never looked back."

Didn't the abrupt change produce digestive problems? "Only briefly," Winkler said. "Every time I introduced a new meat, they would have loose stools for a day or two, but after that their systems adjusted and they were fine." The new foods included not only chicken, venison, beef, lamb, turkey, duck, and rabbit, but also pork, a food few veterinarians recommend. "There's no doubt that it's harder to digest," Winkler said, "and it affected all of my dogs when they first had it, but now they eat pork neck bones with no problem. I feed whatever's available, and they get a constantly changing variety. The only bones I stay away from are big, heavy shank bones. I stick with smaller bones that they can crunch up and eat."

Consider each pet individually and introduce new foods as quickly or as slowly as the animal accepts them. Dogs and cats making the transition from canned or packaged food often are helped by the use of digestive enzymes, acidophilus, and other supplements.

As a general rule, it is easier to introduce new foods to young rather than old animals, and some breeds are more adventurous than others. As much as he liked raw meat, my husband's first red tabby, Pumpkin, loved corn, persimmons, and broccoli. Pumpkin II is fond of dates, avocado, and pecans. Samantha will eat just about everything except citrus fruit and raw mushrooms. Pepper prefers raw poultry and fish, but like our other pets, she is always offered a taste of whatever we're preparing.

A few cats and dogs would rather starve than eat a new food. If an animal doesn't become sufficiently interested in a new food at least to try it, dinnertime becomes a source of stress for both the animal and her owner. Healthy adult dogs and cats can fast for several days without ill effects, but prolonged fasting usually is not recommended, and an animal that goes on a hunger strike faces unknown risks. If your dog or cat is not at all interested in raw meat, raw bones, or other raw foods, continue feeding whatever the animal will eat, but add a tiny amount of fresh, raw meat in the middle. If necessary, grind or puree the meat. If your cat will accept ⅛ of a teaspoon this week, perhaps she will accept ¼ teaspoon next week, and so on. Start with raw meat, the most important ingredient, and deal with bones and other extras later. In time, you should be able to use the original food as a flavoring agent and then discontinue its use altogether.

All pets experience detoxification as their bodies eliminate stored toxins, and in some cases the switch to raw foods coincides with skin bumps, rashes, coat irritations, dreadful-smelling breath, malodorous stools, and other unpleasant symptoms. Herbs and nutritional supplements can help ease these symptoms, but if the animal is reasonably healthy, time alone will repair this temporary condition. Dietary changes usually are easier for younger animals and those in good health than for older pets or those in poor health. If your dog or cat has a serious illness, consult a holistic veterinarian before changing the animal's diet. Many chronic and serious illnesses have been slowed, reversed, or cured by a natural diet introduced by a caring owner with the encouragement of a knowledgeable health care practitioner, but too-rapid detoxification puts a serious strain on the body's organs. A too-rapid shift may be followed by vomiting, diarrhea, and other obvious symptoms. For detoxification support, see pages 94–98 and 203–208.

Commercial Pet Foods

When it comes to convenience, nothing matches commercial pet foods. You don't have to think, plan, organize, refrigerate, or prepare anything. All you do is open a can, box, or bag.

No book about pet nutrition would be complete without a closer look at America's pet foods. Warning: The following may raise your blood pressure and keep you away from supermarket pet food aisles. It certainly will make you a suspicious label reader.

The Bad News

Pet food manufacturers claim that their products are nutritionally balanced and provide 100 percent of everything animals need for good health. The history of commercial pet foods, however, has been marked by tragedies resulting from vitamin, mineral, and other deficiencies. "It wasn't long ago that cat owners were told not to give their pets anything except commercial cat food," says breeder Jo Forsythe, "but it turned out to be deficient in the amino acid taurine. Without taurine, cats develop heart and eye diseases, and a lot of cats died before anyone realized why. Cats on a raw-meat diet get plenty of taurine, and so do dogs. Because today's pet food industry doesn't supplement dog foods with extra taurine, some people wonder whether the growing incidence of heart problems and eye diseases in dogs might be linked to its absence from commercial foods. There's just too much difference between the natural components of raw ingredients and even the best commercial foods to rule out this possibility."

Another concern Forsythe shares with animal nutritionists is the use of hormones in widely used pet food ingredients such as chicken. "There are well-documented endocrine disorders in children who eat large quantities of hormone-treated chicken," she states, "and who knows whether the thyroid problems and other endocrine imbalances now common in dogs and cats have a similar cause?" By feeding poultry and meat grown without hormones and antibiotics, owners can protect their pets from drug residues.

Of greater concern is quality, for very few manufacturers use ingredients suitable for human consumption. Instead, their products are made entirely or mostly from ingredients that are unfit for humans or that are inedible residues left over from the manufacturing and packaging of processed foods. For example, rancid grease collected from restaurants in 50-gallon drums goes to rendering plants for use in pet foods, because this potentially carcinogenic waste product has a fragrance that dogs and cats find attractive.

Here in the United States, feathers, beaks, hooves, horns, diseased tissue, and cancerous tumors all count as pet food protein. Seeing "guaranteed nutritional analysis" on the label tells you nothing about the source of the product's ingredients. Manufacturers are allowed to use 4-D meats, which are rejected for human consumption because the animals they came from were dead, diseased, dying, or disabled on arrival at the slaughterhouse. Animal meal, a primary pet food ingredient, can legally contain ground feathers, nails, claws, cartilage, tendons, bones, blood, and fecal waste. These are of course natural ingredients and exactly what a carnivore devours when eating prey, but the wild carnivore consumes these body parts fresh, raw, and with significant quantities of muscle meat, not after sterilization at high heat in combination with other questionable ingredients.

In 1983, the Pet Food Institute convinced the U.S. Food and Drug Administration (FDA) to allow changes on pet food labels so that cheese rinds could be called cheese, corn husks and peanut shells could be called vegetable fiber, hydrolyzed chicken feathers could be called poultry protein products, and ground bones could be called processed animal protein. The Humane Society of the United States and the American Holistic Veterinary Medical Association strongly opposed the changes because they disguise and misrepresent ingredients.

Animals in the 4-D category are denatured before being sent to rendering plants. Denaturing is any process that makes a substance so unpalatable that no one will consume it. High-proof grain alcohol is denatured before being sold at low cost for external application; the result smells and tastes so terrible that no one is tempted to drink it, thus protecting state and federal alcohol tax revenues. The denaturing of diseased and contaminated meat is a similar process designed to protect human health. If 4-D carcasses were left undisturbed, they probably would find their way to market, but denatured meat is so obviously tainted that no one tries to sell it as food for people. As Wendell O. Belfield, D.V.M., reported in "A Gruesome Account of Food Not Fit for a Pet" in the May 1992 *Let's Live* magazine, the denaturing materials approved by federal meat inspection regulations include fuel oil, kerosene, crude carbolic acid, and citronella. Belfield was a veterinary meat inspector for the U.S. Department of Agriculture and the state of California for seven years, and he saw firsthand the chemical treatment of condemned carcasses sent to rendering plants. Even if charcoal is used for denaturing, no amount of activated charcoal can disguise inferior ingredients, and charcoal is not recommended for daily consumption by any pet.

Because dead animals may be stored without refrigeration for several days before being rendered or processed, their carcasses are often contaminated with *Salmonella, E. Coli* and other bacteria that produce endotoxins. These poisons, which cause disease and are generally harmful to all body tissues, are released when the bacterial cell is broken down or dies and disintegrates. Although the bacteria that release them are destroyed by high-temperature sterilization, the endotoxins are unaffected by heat.

In February of 1990, the *San Francisco Chronicle* printed two articles by investigative reporter John Eckhouse documenting questionable ingredients in pet foods. The articles raised a storm of controversy and indignant denials by pet food industry executives, but the facts are as Eckhouse stated. Federal and state agencies, including the FDA, the American Veterinary Medical Association, state veterinary organizations, and humane societies throughout the United States, confirm that dogs, cats, and other pets are routinely rendered after they die in animal shelters or are disposed of by health authorities, and the end product, labeled tallow, meat meal, or bone meal, serves as raw material for pet foods. According to veterinary researchers quoted by Eckhouse, many of these dead pets were given the euthanizing drug sodium pentobarbital, which is not removed or altered by the rendering process. In addition to containing trace amounts of this drug, rendered products are preserved with chemicals such as BHA (butylated hydroxyanisole) and BHT (butylated hydroxytoluene), both known to cause kidney and liver dysfunction. Their use is prohibited in several European countries. Ethoxyquin, another fat stabilizer in common use, has been the subject of many articles in holistic pet magazines. It is a suspected carcinogen and has been linked with a number of possible health problems in animals.

Most commercially raised cattle, sheep, and other grass-eating animals are fed supplements containing protein rendered from diseased livestock. This agricultural practice, which is widespread in the United States and England, is described in the article "Could Mad-Cow Disease Happen Here?" by Ellen Ruppel Shell in the September 1998 *Atlantic Monthly*. Research has shown that illnesses specific to one species can spread to others when animals are forced to consume each other's diseased tissue. Shell criticized the U.S. Department of Agriculture for not outlawing the rendering of neurological material and infectious material from cattle and other animals, for their agricultural use poses a potential, if indirect, risk to human consumers. She didn't mention the far greater risk rendered products pose to pets who consume them directly.

Although trace amounts of pharmaceutical drugs, pesticides, endotoxins, toxic chemicals, lead, and other contaminants in commercial pet foods may not cause the dramatic symptoms of acute poisoning, their cumulative effects can be detrimental to any animal. Pets being weaned from commercial pet foods in favor of a raw, natural diet usually benefit from the daily use of foods, supplements, and herbs such as those described on pages 203–208, which support detoxification.

The Good News

Aren't there any "good" pet foods on the market? Better foods are available today than ten years ago, but no commercial food equals the biologically appropriate natural diet you can prepare at home.

If your dog or cat will accept a new type of kibble but will not yet accept raw meaty bones, you can compare labels and use, as a transition diet, foods that contain human food-grade meat or poultry, a minimum amount of grain (preferably none), no tallow, no meat meal or bone meal (the rendered products that contain deceased dogs and cats), no artificial flavors or colors, and no chemical preservatives. If it's canned or packaged, the food probably will have been heated above body temperature, killing its enzymes and heat-sensitive nutrients. Although you can add enzymes and other supplements to help your pet digest and assimilate this food, it will not contain everything its raw ingredients contained, and it won't contain the whole raw bones that dogs and cats need for pefect health. If it's frozen, it will be made of ground meat, not the large chunks and whole pieces that dogs and cats need to chew on for good dental health and stomach exercise, and if it contains bones, they will be ground, too. If it's freeze-dried, it's likely to be made of ground beef, like Solid Gold's Buckaroo Beef. This convenience food from free-range cattle is far superior to commercial pet foods, but it is not a substitute for a well-balanced raw diet.

In addition, most frozen pet foods contain synthetic vitamins and other questionable ingredients because commercial diets are designed to be "balanced." Some popular products consist of grains and supplement powders to which you add raw meat and vegetables, which is a step in the right direction. It makes more sense, though, to start with the raw meaty bones your pet needs, leave out the grain, and add a changing variety of extras.

The Bottom Line

As hundreds of dog and cat lovers have discovered after juggling complicated schedules of supplements and different types of canned or kibble pet food, the easiest way to feed your pet is with raw meaty bones and table scraps.

The only canned or packaged pet food I know of that has not been damaged by high-heat processing is BalanceDiet. Although not raw, this brand of dog and cat food (see Resources) is made of USDA meat, poultry, fish, and eggs, plus vegetables and other whole foods in a fermentation process that retains their enzymes and other "live" nutrients. Some who feed a bone-based raw diet use BalanceDiet for convenience while traveling, in emergencies, and as a supplement for pets requiring extra nutrition.

The Fine Art of Stool Watching

One of the simplest ways to monitor your pet's digestion is to keep careful track of what he or she eats—and to monitor what comes out the other end.

As your dog moves from grain-based, canned, or packaged food to more natural fare, the most significant difference you will notice is the great reduction in stool size. Healthy stools are firm, compact, and well shaped. Dogs on a bone-based raw diet seldom if ever have anal sac problems, for these glands and the muscles around them are well exercised. Depending on the supplements and vegetables you add, stools may be colorful—grass green, for example, or carrot orange.

You may notice mucus-covered stools as bone residue is eliminated. As Richard Pitcairn warns, too much raw bone too soon can cause temporary problems in a dog whose digestive tract has been weakened by cooked, canned, or packaged foods. This reaction decreases as the animal's system adjusts and is unlikely to recur in dogs that are fed raw bones daily or several times per week.

Obviously, diarrhea is a warning sign. In many cases, it is a temporary, self-correcting condition, but diarrhea that doesn't disappear within one day is a cause for concern. It may be caused by a specific food, which is why food diaries are important in the diagnosis of allergies and food sensitivities. Keep track of what your dog eats and, if loose stools always follow a certain food, eliminate that food and see if the problem disappears.

The fecal matter of other animals deserves attention, too. Dogs are notorious for eating manure, goose droppings, cat litter offerings, and even their own stools, a condition called *coprophagia*. Although it is usually considered a behavioral problem, coprophagia is probably nutritional. Dogs fed a well-balanced natural diet are less likely to eat their own feces than dogs fed commercial pet foods. Adding mineral-rich supplements such as kelp often breaks them of this habit. The consumption of substances that are not foods is called pica, a related condition; see page 69.

Still, even the best-fed dogs may go out of their way to find cow, horse, sheep, or goose manure. Is this habit disgusting or healthy or what? Juliette de Bairacli Levy encourages dogs to enjoy these delicacies as long as they come from vegetarian animals. Manure contains large quantities of active bacteria, enzymes, minerals, and other nutrients. Many holistic veterinarians agree, especially those who keep livestock or who grew up on farms. It may not be appetizing to humans, but neither you nor your pet is likely to contract any illness or infection from your pet's occasional indulgence.

Pets as Vegetarians

Food is the social cement that binds us together as families and cultures. It excites our passions. Some of us devote our lives to food: We grow it, sell it, study it, prepare it, teach people what to eat or how to eat, write about it, and publish books about it. Everyone talks about food. It's something we deal with every day. People argue, debate, discuss, and even fight about food. If we worry about our own diets, the feeding of our children and pets is no doubt fraught with anxiety and conflicting opinions. In the world of dog people, food is as emotional an issue as crates and pinch collars.

Most American dog owners will never feed their pets a raw diet. They believe canned or packaged food is what dogs are supposed to eat, and people who do weird things like feed their pets raw bones are just asking for trouble. A smaller group is experimenting with raw diets and telling anyone who will listen about their spectacular results. An even smaller group is experimenting with vegetarian diets for dogs and cats, and they, too, are encouraging others to follow their example.

In the late 1980s, when I began considering a raw diet for our cats, I had been a strict vegan for years. Vegans are vegetarians who don't use anything that comes from animals, including fish, poultry, eggs, milk, or honey. I'd spent most of my adult life fielding the questions of concerned meat-eaters who worried that my health must be suffering, so going without meat was not an unfamiliar concept. But the nutritional needs of cats are so different from those of people that the task of creating a balanced, healthy menu for them seemed formidable. In the end, Francis Pottenger's experiments convinced me that raw is better than cooked, and Mother Nature is the best guide.

There are political, religious, and philosophical reasons for pursuing a vegetarian diet, but do they apply to our nonvegetarian companion animals? To my knowledge, no spiritual or religious leader has ever suggested that dogs or cats be deprived of meat, for doing so would violate the laws of nature.

Some have argued that dogs can be vegetarians without much trouble, but cats, who are true carnivores, cannot. It's true that dogs can survive on vegetarian fare, but do they thrive? The supplements that would benefit vegetarian dogs—cold-sterilized bone meal, glandular concentrates, fish oils, and whole-food extracts containing liver and other organs—come from animal sources and are therefore inappropriate. It is a dilemma.

In the end, each owner makes a personal choice, and that choice must be respected. I hope all those who live with a dog or cat will let thousands of years of natural selection define their canine and feline menu planning. If that isn't possible, I hope they will do whatever they can within the constraints of their philosophy to provide the nutrition their animals require. After all is said and done, love is probably the most important ingredient in any animal's life.

Chapter 2

Supplements for Pets

D
ogs and cats that are born to healthy parents who ate a well-balanced raw diet and who are themselves fed this way don't need much in the way of nutritional supplements. Unfortunately, hardly any of America's pets fit that description. This chapter describes several of the numerous supplements that help dogs and cats improve their digestion and maintain good health. The food supplement business is bewilderingly large, but the following are among the most widely recommended for use with pets.

The Importance of Enzymes

Enzymes are proteins that in small amounts speed the rate of biological reactions such as digestion. Unstable and easily inactivated by heat and certain chemicals, enzymes are produced within living cells to perform specific biochemical reactions. Nearly every raw food contains the enzymes necessary for its digestion, but cooking inactivates these enzymes and the body must work hard to replace them in order for food to be broken down and assimilated.

Coenzymes are nonprotein substances that combine with protein to form a complete enzyme. Most of the coenzymes important in human, canine, and feline nutrition are produced from vitamins or are themselves vitamins. Lipoic acid, once thought to be a member of the B-complex vitamins, and coenzyme Q10, which resembles vitamin E, are popular supplements because they help prevent and treat chronic illnesses. For example, lipoic acid, which is abundant in red meat, is a powerful antioxidant that removes toxins from the body, helps prevent cataracts, increases immune function, and improves the health of nerves. In animal studies, 100 milligrams of lipoic acid per kilogram of body weight improved memory. Coenzyme Q10, another important antioxidant, has been used to treat cancer, improve respiratory function, heal ulcers, prevent allergies, and improve heart health in humans and animals. Mackerel, salmon, and sardines are the leading food sources of coenzyme Q10. Like food enzymes, coenzymes deteriorate at temperatures above approximately 115 degrees F.

For those unable to provide an all-raw diet for their pets, enzyme supplements replace at least some of the enzymes killed by the cooking and processing of food. Enzyme supplements can be added to raw foods, too, especially for dogs and cats that previously have been fed a commercial diet, are recovering from an illness, have been treated with antibiotics, or experience any digestive difficulty. Enzyme supplements (see the Resources for this chapter at the back of this book) have impressive records of safety and health improvement for animals of every description, from dogs, cats, and horses to reptiles, birds, fish, primates, and humans. The addition of enzymes to processed food improves digestion and assimilation so effectively that the quantity of food may have to be reduced by 15 to 20 percent to prevent unwanted weight gain. Veterinarians who have tested enzyme supplements report improved coats, uniform litters, higher puppy survival rates, fewer problems in pregnancy, and increased mobility in older dogs, including improvement in hip dysplasia, all without vitamin or mineral supplementation. Enzymes increase the assimilation of vitamins, minerals, and other nutrients.

Plant-derived enzymes include protease, which digests protein; lipase, which digests fats; and amylase, which digests starch or carbohydrates. When taken on an empty stomach, these enzymes reduce inflammation, improve immune function, and stimulate the digestion of bacteria, toxins, and partly digested proteins. Papain, derived from papaya, has anti-inflammatory and wound-healing properties. Bromelain, derived from pineapple, reduces inflammation and helps prevent bruising.

Antioxidant enzymes, found in fresh sprouts, convert potentially damaging free radicals to harmless oxygen and water. The best known antioxidant enzymes are superoxide dismutase (SOD), catalase, glutathione peroxidase, and methionine reductase.

Pancreatic enzymes usually are derived from the pancreas of cattle. Pancreatin works only in the small intestine. Given with food, it assists in the digestion of protein, fats, and carbohydrates, and it can prevent adverse food reactions. Consumed on an empty stomach, it reduces inflammation and pain throughout the body and helps eliminate intestinal parasites by literally digesting them.

According to Nancy Scanlan, D.V.M., enzyme deficiencies cause coprophagia in some dogs (see page 53). "Sometimes dogs don't produce enough digestive enzymes," she said in a June 1998 *Whole Dog Journal* interview. "It seems curious, but these dogs are compelled to eat their feces because it contains the digestive enzymes they need—a kind of disgusting recycling system." In addition to supplying all the minerals a dog requires (stool eating is often linked with mineral deficiencies), feeding foods rich in enzymes can help prevent coprophagia.

You don't need a product labeled "enzymes" to supply these vital nutrients to your pet. All growing sprouts, grasses, and herbs contain them. Sprouting authority Victor Vulkinskas often described how his mentor, the late Ann Wigmore of wheat grass fame, improved the health of her animals with live foods. Wigmore's chickens and rabbits doubled in size when she gave them enzyme-rich wheat sprouts; an underweight, ulcerated monkey regained its health on wheat sprouts; and her cats showed dramatic improvements in behavior and appearance whenever wheat grass and sprouting wheat were added to their commercial pet food.

While visiting his parents, Vulkinskas was dismayed to see that the family's Pekingese dog, which had been fed rich table scraps for five years, was now suffering from spinal problems due to cancerous growths that prevented the use of his hind legs. Because there was no hope of recovery, the veterinarian recommended euthanasia. Vulkinskas mixed powdered wheat grass juice with water, and the dog lapped it up. "To my surprise," he said, "the following morning he was waiting for me with a big grin at my second-floor bedroom door and leaped into the air trying to lick my face—an amazing feat even for a healthy Pekingese!" The dog lived another five years and always begged for the green powder whenever he and Vulkinskas shared a meal.

"All the literature I have explored in the field of enzymes are based on studies with experimental animals," Vulkinskas said, "and the results are consistent. Enzyme-rich diets promote recovery, reduce the incidence of disease, and improve the quality of life."

Although most plants are rich sources of enzymes, a few, primarily raw seeds and nuts, contain enzyme inhibitors. Give seeds and nuts in small quantities, feed them to your pet with an enzyme supplement, or for best results, sprout seeds and soak nuts overnight to inactivate their enzyme inhibitors.

Vitamins

Vitamins are substances required in small amounts for healthy growth and development. Because they cannot be synthesized in the body, they are essential constituents of the diet. Vitamins are divided into two groups. The water-soluble group includes the B-complex vitamins, vitamin C, and bioflavonoids, which are sometimes called vitamin P. The fat-soluble vitamins are A, D, E, and K, all of which are stored in the body, and essential fatty acids, which are sometimes called vitamin F. Lack of sufficient quantities of any of these vitamins or their close relatives manifests as a deficiency disease or some form of impaired health.

Many veterinarians believe supplements are both a waste of money and potentially harmful. Others, such as Wendell Belfield, D.V.M., disagree. Belfield has found that vitamin and mineral supplements make a dramatic difference in the health of dogs and cats. Of course, all of his patients developed their deficiencies eating commercial pet foods. When fresh foods provide all the nutrients an animal needs, supplementation isn't necessary.

In an ideal world, all our animals would be fed as Francis Pottenger's cats, cows, chickens, and guinea pigs were, on fresh, whole, raw foods in fresh air and sunlight. Alas, this is not an ideal world. Unless you provide everything your pet needs from your own bucolic farm or sheep ranch, your dog or cat probably will benefit from occasional supplements, and if your pet has spent a lifetime on commercial pet food, the right vitamins and minerals may save his life.

Vitamin C

Because of nutritional studies conducted shortly after World War II, most veterinarians believe that dogs and cats produce all the vitamin C their bodies need. For this reason it is not an ingredient in pet foods. However, when Belfield began using vitamin C on his canine and feline patients, they responded dramatically. According to Belfield, vitamin C prevents a variety of health problems, including degenerative spine disorders, arthritis, skin and coat conditions, ruptured discs, hip dysplasia—which he considers a subclinical form of scurvy—and feline leukemia. In his books, *The Very Healthy Cat Book* and *How to Have a Healthier Dog*, Belfield devotes long chapters to vitamin C, documenting its ability to improve immunity, treat viral and bacterial infections, detoxify the body, improve collagen, and improve the condition of cancer patients. He also dispels the myth that large quantities of vitimin C can be toxic or cause kidney stones.

For best results, use a natural C-complex vitamin that includes bio-flavonoids. Adult dogs and cats on a raw diet that includes fresh fruits and vegetables don't need large amounts of supplemental C, but the addition of 500 milligrams every few days is inexpensive insurance. If using vita-min C from whole-food sources, smaller doses are effective. Whenever the animal is stressed from overwork, breeding, emotional or physical trauma, surgery, an accident, or illness, give additional amounts of this essential nutrient.

Vitamin A

Vitamin A, a fat-soluble nutrient, is essential for the maintenance of soft mucous tissues, normal growth, and healthy eyes. Deficiencies cause stunted growth, night blindness, and other vision disorders. Beta carotene in foods such as carrots and yams converts to vitamin A in the canine body; animal sources such as cod liver or salmon oil are recom-mended for cats.

B Vitamins

The B-complex vitamins (thiamine, niacin, riboflavin, biotin, folic acid, pan-tothenic acid, and others) are vital to the health of the nervous system. Deficiencies in this group can manifest as symptoms anywhere in the body, most often in the mouth, eyes, and reproductive organs. These are among the most fragile and heat-sensitive vitamins. Like vitamin C, they are water soluble and are not stored in the body. Liver and other organ meats, fish, poultry, brewer's yeast, eggs, beans, peas, dark green leafy vegetables, whole grains, and dairy products are rich sources of B-complex vitamins. Once or twice a week you may want to give your pet a supplement derived from whole-food sources for humans and adjust the dosage to your pet's weight.

Vitamin D

Vitamin D is called the sunshine vitamin because exposure to sunlight manufactures it in the body. Vitamin D, which is also supplied by fatty fish, is necessary for healthy bones. Veterinarians recommend up to 100 International Units (IUs) per 20 pounds of body weight, but half an hour in the summer sun can produce that much and more. According to recent research, winter sunlight in latitudes north of New York City produces no vitamin D, but if exposed to sufficient summer sunlight, the body stores enough for the rest of the year. While excess vitamin D produced by the sun is nontoxic, excessive amounts from supplements are potentially dangerous.

Vitamin E

Vitamin E is essential during every phase of life, including gestation. Animals with high vitamin E levels tend to have stronger, healthier litters and easier birthings than those with low levels. Vitamin E speeds the healing of wounds and burns, improves the assimilation and distribution of nutrients throughout the body, keeps the heart healthy, invigorates older animals, slows the symptoms of aging, protects cats against steatitis (a painful disease of fatty tissue resulting from diets high in the unsaturated fats of fish oils), improves the skin and coats of all animals, and boosts resistance to disease.

Food sources include vegetable oils, nuts, dark green leafy vegetables, organ meats, seafood, eggs, and avocados. Dogs and cats with heart disease, athletic or working dogs, breeding or pregnant animals, and any pet under stress may benefit from supplemental vitamin E. Standard Process Cataplex E-2 is a superior product that can be given in low doses to improve heart function and help prevent disease.

Vitamin K

Vitamin K regulates blood clotting and other clotting factors; it is also essential for kidney function and bone metabolism. Food sources include beef liver, cheese, oats, cabbage, turnip greens, and other dark green leafy vegetables. Healthy animals on a natural diet receive ample amounts of this vitamin.

Bioflavonoids

There are a thousand or more bioflavonoids, which usually occur in combination with vitamin C in leaves, bark, rinds, flowers, and seeds. While bioflavonoids often act as coloring pigments in plants, their more important function for human, feline, and canine nutrition appears to be their synergistic partnership with vitamin C. Citrus fruits are high in hesperidin and eriocitrin, buckwheat is rich in rutin, and other sprouts are rich in quercetin, to name four of the most familiar bioflavonoids.

Antioxidants

Vitamins A, C, and E, bioflavonoids, and the mineral selenium are antioxidants; that is, they protect fatty acids in cells from damaging oxidation by free radicals, which are unstable molecules that damage healthy cells while robbing them of electrons. Belfield has described several chronic illnesses in dogs and cats that responded to antioxidant therapy after conventional treatments such as antibiotics failed. These included ear infections, the gum disease gingivitis, miliary dermatitis, colitis, heart disease (valvular insufficiency), and cancer.

When Wendell Belfield began treating dogs and cats with vitamins, his work created a storm of controversy. How times have changed. Now even conventional veterinarians prescribe vitamins, and the production of supplements for pets has become a worldwide industry. "I am no longer a maverick or nonconformist," he remarked. "I am now mainstream."

Natural Versus Synthetic

In any discussion of supplements, it's necessary to examine the differences between vitamins and other nutrients found in food and their synthetic counterparts made from chemicals. Nobel Prizes have been awarded for vitamin synthesis, the scientific community regards synthetics as identical to natural nutrients, and the low cost of synthetic supplements makes them affordable to all.

But are synthetic and natural nutrients really the same? Their molecular structures may match, but they are not mirror images of each other. Living bodies can tell the difference, and the difference can be debilitating.

In the 1930s, Barnett Sure at the University of Arkansas conducted hundreds of experiments on the links between nutrition and fertility, for it is in their reproduction that animals most dramatically and rapidly manifest nutritional imbalances and deficiencies. Sure's laboratory animals repeatedly showed that supplementation with synthetic B-complex vitamins interfered with normal reproduction, causing lactation problems, sterility, stillbirths, and infant mortality. The more synthetic vitamins his animals ingested, the worse their reproductive health.

Synthetic and natural vitamins interact differently with minerals in the body. For example, many nutritionally oriented physicians, such as *Health Alert* editor Bruce West, M.D., warn their patients and readers not to take ascorbic acid (synthetic vitamin C) because it depletes copper levels. The natural vitamin C in citrus fruits, acerola cherries, amla berries, rose hips, red and green peppers, and other fruits and vegetables does not. In addition, ascorbic acid is only one of many chemicals in the natural vitamin C complex; it really is not vitamin C at all. Some vitamin C supplements are labeled "natural and organic" because they are synthesized from corn sugar (glucose), which technically fits that definition, but they are not the same as a natural vitamin C complex from whole food.

Bioflavonoids such as rutin, quercetin, and hesperidin occur naturally in the pulp and peel of citrus fruits, peppers, buckwheat, black currants, algae, and other plants. Because bioflavonoids enhance the absorption of vitamin C, they are often combined in supplements, but the bioflavonoids in a vitamin C product are as likely to be synthetic as the vitamin C itself.

Antioxidant supplements are a big business, and in addition to the well-known combination of selenium and vitamins A, C, and E, antioxidants such as beta carotene, lycopene, lutein, coenzyme Q10, alpha lipoic acid, and proanthocyanidins are sold separately. When beta carotene failed to protect heavy smokers from heart attacks, headlines condemned vitamin therapies without noting that the supplement tested was synthetic and not derived from food.

Critics of isolated nutrients note that taking beta carotene by itself no matter what its source is unnatural, for foods rich in beta carotene contain other nutrients that work synergistically to protect health. For example, spirulina contains alpha carotene, beta carotene, zeaxanthin, cryptoxanthin, and other carotenes. Among their other benefits, mixed carotenoids have been shown to protect the skin against the harmful effects of ultraviolet radiation and reduce DNA damage, a leading cause of cancer. Carrots are another rich source of carotenes, containing alpha carotene, beta carotene, epsilon carotene, gamma carotene, lycopene, and dozens of compounds that have yet to be identified. As David G. Williams, M.D., wrote in the August 1996 edition of his *Alternatives* newsletter, "It would be a serious mistake to think that a single beta carotene supplement would provide the same protection as the combination of carotenes found in carrots."

In response to the increasing demand for natural or food-based vitamins, more manufacturers are supplying them. Labels are not always easy to decipher, however. If a label uses the abbreviation USP for United States Pharmacopoeia, this assurance of purity is also an indication that the nutrient was manufactured from chemicals, not from whole foods. Sustained-release or timed-release products are always synthetic, and any label showing that the supplement provides a substantial vitamin dose almost always indicates a synthetic product. If a label advertises nutrients "such as are found in whole foods," they may not come from whole foods. Check the ingredients or contact the manufacturer.

Americans have become so accustomed to megadose vitamin therapies that the labels of Standard Process supplements (see Resources), which are derived from whole foods, look like misprints. Cataplex E-2 tablets contain only 2 IUs of vitamin E, and the recommended human maintenance dose is two tablets per day. The Wysong product Food-C contains 150 milligrams vitamin C per capsule and Nature's Plus brand of chewable Acerola-C Complex (available in health food stores) contains 250 milligrams vitamin C per wafer, whereas synthetic supplements of the same size contain six to eight times those amounts. How can such small doses make a difference to you or your pet?

The answer lies in how our bodies recognize and process nutrients in food (which are familiar and easily assimilated) in contrast to our very different response to synthetic or fractionated supplements. Made from glandular materials, high-selenium yeast, and calcium, Cataplex E-2 is the most popular Standard Process product, best known for its ability to improve cardiac function, prevent heart arrhythmia and angina, increase the distribution of oxygen throughout the respiratory system, increase stamina, and help prevent infection. Given at the rate of 1 tablet every other day for cats and small dogs, 1 tablet per day for medium dogs, and 2 tablets per day for large dogs, Cataplex E-2 helps prevent reproductive problems, maintain heart health, promote efficient detoxification, and improve endurance.

Wysong's Food-C contains sprouted barley, acerola juice, black currants, grape juice, whole rice syrup, rose hips, composted kelp, orange juice, barley grass juice, wheat grass juice, sea plant (*S. platensis*), and blue algae. Instead of a single vitamin, Food-C contains more than 115 nutrients, including vitamins, minerals, enzymes, bioflavonoids, antioxidants, and essential fatty acids. Nature's Plus Acerola-C Complex contains acerola extract powder, lemon bioflavonoid complex, rose hip extract, black currant concentrate, green pepper extract, and rutin from natural sources, making it another easily assimilated source of related nutrients.

Many excellent supplements make no claims of specific potency. The Vitamin Shoppe's Green Phyters tablets (see Resources) contain organically grown, freeze-dried spirulina, chlorella, barley juice, wheat grass, and alfalfa leaf. Wysong's Salad capsules contain extracts and concentrates of broccoli, Brussels sprouts, cauliflower, red and green cabbage, kale, and broccoli sprouts. Neither product claims to contain any measured amount of any nutrient, but both are superior to synthetic supplements of guaranteed potency.

Whole-food supplements are so different from synthetics that label comparisons can be meaningless. More is not necessarily better, and although large doses of synthetic vitamins have been used with much success in the treatment of malnourished dogs and cats, megavitamins not only are unnecessary for perfect health, but they also can cause nutritional imbalances and have adverse side effects.

Minerals

Since the late 1800s, America's farm soils have been stripped by modern farming methods of their minerals and trace elements. The result is such a severe depletion that the mineral levels of our industrially grown staple crops are insufficient to provide and maintain good health. The most widely used chemical fertilizers contain only two or three minerals, not the seventy-two or more trace elements found in nature.

Mineral deficiencies interfere with vitamin absorption, digestion, and the health of every body system, from the brain's electrical circuitry to the healthy operation of the heart, circulatory system, reproductive organs, skeleton, skin, lungs, and everything else. A lifetime of health problems can be prevented by feeding puppies, kittens, and other young animals the minerals their growing bodies require.

In the May 1996 *Journal of the American Holistic Veterinary Medical Association*, Martin Schulman, V.M.D., reported that mineral deficiencies often contribute to the development of seizures in dogs. In his clinic, a review of the medical histories of canines diagnosed with epilepsy revealed that an "astonishingly high percentage" showed significant manifestations of pica, an eating disorder caused by malnutrition. In one case, a female German Shepherd Dog had a history of licking wrought iron and eating glass and Christmas tree lights. An improved diet supplemented with plant-derived colloidal minerals, digestive enzymes, and probiotic foods cured the pica within three weeks and the dog had no additional seizures.

Seaweeds such as kelp and dulse provide dozens of minerals, including iodine. Brazil nuts are rich in selenium. Blackstrap molasses and wheat germ contain substantial amounts of magnesium. Fruits, nuts, and vegetables are rich in boron. Kelp, nuts, and seeds are sources of chromium. Avocados and fish are rich in copper. Deep-sea fish contain iodine. Organ meats provide substantial amounts of iron and potassium. Raw meaty bones offer calcium, copper, chromium, magnesium, phosphorus, manganese, molybdenum, sulfur, vanadium, zinc, and other minerals in perfect balance; bone marrow is rich in copper and iron. Unrefined sea salt (see page 76) contains trace amounts of all of nature's minerals.

The advantage to food-derived minerals is that they are easy to assimilate in proportions that living bodies utilize well. Ian Billinghurst based his dogs' diet on bones because they provide a puppy's most complete and balanced supply of minerals, preventing hip dysplasia, growth defects, wobbler syndrome, dropped hocks, and bone cysts. "We have been breeding Great Danes and Rottweilers for years," he explains. "The bone problems our dogs had been experiencing disappeared the moment we began to raise our puppies on a bone-based diet." The larger the breed, Billinghurst cautions, the more important it is not to use calcium supplements. These supplements have been shown to disrupt the balance of minerals needed by the body and exacerbate bone and growth problems.

Whenever providing a mineral supplement, consider using a liquid or powder that contains most or all of the elements found in nature rather than a product that contains only one, two, or five minerals. Mineral supplements derived from plant material, ocean water, or salt lakes are easily absorbed, well tolerated, and in natural balance. These sources have been called dangerous because they contain small quantities of aluminum, arsenic, cadmium, lead, mercury, and other toxic elements. Although the microscopic amounts in unrefined sea salt have never been shown to affect human or animal health adversely, some manufacturers of concentrated colloidal minerals remove potentially toxic minerals and trace elements from their products.

The claim that plant-derived minerals do not accumulate in the body is supported by research on kelp, some species of which are known for their high arsenic content. Elemental arsenic accumulates in the body, and it doesn't take much of it to kill a human, but plant-derived arsenic behaves differently. In Japan, which has the world's highest per capita consumption of kelp, tests on human volunteers showed that 100 percent of the arsenic ingested in seaweed was excreted in the urine within sixty hours. In addition to correcting mineral deficiencies, kelp and other seaweeds contain alginates that soothe and cleanse the digestive tract while preventing the absorption of toxic metals including mercury, cadmium, cesium, plutonium, strontium, and other radioactive isotopes.

Amino Acids

Amino acids are the building blocks of proteins needed to construct every cell of every organ, bone, and fluid in the body. Eight are called essential amino acids because they cannot be synthesized by the body and must be supplied in food or supplements, and the remaining fourteen, called nonessential acids, are formed within the body by essential amino acids. For optimum health, essential amino acids must be provided in the proper balance. Amino acids are sold separately or in blends as nutritional powders or capsules. Label directions usually recommend that they be taken between meals on an empty stomach.

Dogs and cats on a well-balanced raw diet receive ample amino acids. Supplemental amino acids are recommended for pets that have been eating a commercial diet (processing destroys fragile amino acids) or are recovering from a serious illness.

L-taurine, manufactured in the body by methionine and cysteine, corrects the composition of bile, helps regulate blood sugar levels, keeps the heart muscle strong, and improves eye function. Deficiencies are considered a possible cause of epilepsy. Taurine is essential to all mammals, especially cats, which evolved on a taurine-rich diet. When commercial pet foods contained insufficient taurine, many cats died of heart failure. The taurine content of a typical mouse (2.4 milligrams per gram) is more than ten times that of most foods your indoor pet is likely to encounter, including beef (.2 milligram), beef liver (.1 milligram), chicken (.2 milligram), eggs (.1 milligram), and milk (.05 milligram). Clams are high in taurine (1 milligram per gram). There is no significant vegetable source of this amino acid.

Raw meat, bones, and eggs are excellent sources of amino acids. A dog or cat eating a well-balanced raw diet receives all the amino acids needed for good health. Holistic veterinarians sometimes prescribe amino acid supplements for pets that have been fed commercial pet food or a home-prepared diet of cooked food, especially if they suffer from digestive problems or a chronic illness. In pets of all ages, amino acids are essential for efficient detoxification (see page 96). One excellent whole-food source of amino acids is the supplement Seacure (see page 90).

Essential Fatty Acids

Essential fatty acids, or EFAs, are the building blocks of fats. Omega-6 linoleic and omega-3 alpha-linoleic acids cannot be manufactured by the body; they must be supplied by foods or supplements. Avocados are an excellent source of "good" fats, especially when accompanied by unrefined sea salt, which, according to biochemist Jacques de Langre, improves the oil's assimilation. Many dogs and a surprising number of cats adore avocados.

Safflower and corn oil are high in linoleic acid, an important unsaturated fatty acid, but for every vote in favor of safflower oil, there is one against it because of its omega-3–omega-6 fatty acid imbalance. Cats don't metabolize unsaturated fats as well as dogs do because of their more restricted carnivorous diet. Pottenger's cats thrived on cod liver oil. Several holistic veterinarians report good results from feeding both dogs and cats a changing assortment of vegetable and animal oils, such as flaxseed, olive, corn, wheat germ, salmon, and cod liver oil as well as raw butter from organically raised cattle.

Although flaxseed oil is so popular that some pet owners feed it as their animals' only significant source of fat, vegetable oils do not contain all of the vitamins found in fish oils or raw butter. In feeding experiments, dogs receiving only flaxseed oil and commercial pet food suffered from bone and skeletal problems. When fish oil replaced the flaxseed oil, these problems disappeared. While vegetable oils are important sources of essential fatty acids, a well-balanced raw diet for dogs and cats includes ample fats and oils from animal sources as well.

Rancidity is a serious problem in fats and oils. To avoid it, keep oils refrigerated. Rancid oils destroy biotin and vitamin E, and the fats in meat and meat by-products are often rancid even before they are used in processed pet foods. Dry pet foods stored for long periods are another source of rancid fats. Obviously, an animal eating a well-prepared home diet never encounters rancidity.

EFA supplements are used to treat and prevent skin and coat conditions, splitting claws or nails, heart disease, hormone imbalances, cancer, and diabetes. The most popular omega-6 supplements are made from the seeds of evening primrose, borage, and black currant; common sources of omega-3 oils include flaxseed and fish oils. Other important sources of EFAs include nuts and seeds.

Gamma-linoleic acid, or GLA, another essential fatty acid, is found in evening primrose and other oils. GLA supports the body's production of hormones known as prostaglandins, which affect hormone balance.

Hormones and Glandular Extracts

In the wild, dogs and cats don't dine on just rib steaks and drumsticks. The first things most foxes, coyotes, wolves, hyenas, feral dogs, lions, tigers, and even domestic cats eat are the prey's digestive organs. Then they consume all the other organs and glands, including the thymus, spleen, brain, eyes, thyroid, pituitary, and adrenals. Glands contain hormones, which are substances that travel through the bloodstream to distant organs and tissues modifying their structures and functions. For example, hormones play an important role in the growth of new skin and hair; they keep black noses black and pink noses pink, prevent fur from changing color, intensify coat color, and help prevent allergic reactions.

Although all of the glands in the body serve an essential purpose, the thymus is called the master gland, or the "seat" of the immune system. It produces various hormonelike substances that affect the maturation and growth of T-cells, which are crucial to the body's defense against cancer and other illnesses. Whole-thymus extracts and products derived from thymus gland tissue, such as thymic protein, have been used to enhance immunity during the treatment of all types of illnesses in dogs and cats as well as people. Hepatitis and other liver diseases often respond quickly to thymus supplements; in fact, thymus extract has cured many chronic human cases of hepatitis within a few weeks.

The adrenal glands lie on top of the kidneys. Their secretions regulate metabolism and maintain the balance of sodium and potassium in the blood. Older animals, animals on a commercial diet, and animals under stress often suffer from adrenal gland exhaustion or depletion.

The pancreas, an organ as well as a gland, is located behind and slightly below the stomach; its most important function is to produce insulin, the hormone that breaks down sugars. Diabetes, an increasingly common illness in commercially fed animals, results from insufficient insulin production.

In the brain, the pineal gland releases melatonin, the hormone that maintains the body's daily rhythms, and the pituitary gland releases hormones that control other endocrine glands. In the throat, the parathyroid gland activates bone-destroying cells, which release calcium into the blood, and the thyroid gland regulates metabolic rate and body temperature. Hypothyroid (underactive thyroid) conditions are common in dogs, and hyperthyroid (overactive thyroid) conditions are common in cats.

Sex-specific hormones, including estrogen in females and testosterone in males, have a direct effect on reproductive organs and an indirect effect on other organs and systems throughout the body.

The few people who feed their dogs and cats glandular supplements claim excellent results. Glandulars are not a quick fix. They require months of daily supplementation to make a difference, but they correct imbalances as no other nutrients can. These are among the easiest supplements to administer, for dogs and cats actively seek them out. I learned this when the Pet Friends Company sent samples of Pet GO glandular wafers for a dog nutrition workshop I was scheduled to give at the home of my friend Sarah Wilson. Samantha, my Labrador Retriever, escorted the sealed box from the front door to the kitchen, sniffing enthusiastically and begging for a taste of whatever might be inside. Each sample consisted of two glandular wafers in a small plastic bag stapled to an information card. I left three of the samples at home and took the rest to Sarah's house, where I put them in an upstairs bedroom with other workshop materials. I was followed by several eager cats and dogs who wanted a taste. When I returned home, I discovered that our cat Pepper had ripped open all three packages, and Sarah reported that the samples at her house had been similarly raided. This was the first time we had seen such a dramatic reaction in not one but all of our pets. It convinced us that glandular extracts supply important nutrients that are missing from the normal fare of dogs and cats, even when they're fed an all-raw diet.

For best results, animal nutritionist Marina Zacharias suggests having a complete blood panel done to test hormone levels and other factors to determine which supplements would be most effective. If the animal has no apparent health problems, providing a variety of glandular supplements from organically raised, minimally processed sources on a rotating basis will supply the nutrients otherwise missing from a pet's food. Supplements made from whole glands, usually derived from cattle, contain little if any active hormones but supply unique nutrients.

Other Helpful Supplements

Kelp and Other Seaweeds

Best known for their abundant minerals and trace elements, kelp and other sea vegetables have a nourishing and tonic effect on all of the body's systems. In the 1930s, Juliette de Bairacli Levy was the first in the West to recommend kelp as a nutritional supplement for animals. Her suggestion was greeted with scorn from the veterinary world, but opinions have changed and kelp is now widely used.

In addition to correcting mineral deficiencies, kelp and other seaweeds contain alginates that soothe and cleanse the digestive tract, improve glandular function, promote rapid hair growth, and correct pigmentation, making black fur and noses truly black. They are important for healthy reproduction and protect against heart and kidney disease. For information on seaweed's safety, see pages 69–70.

Any sea vegetable can be added to your pet's food. Most health food stores offer a variety of North American and Japanese seaweeds, such as nori, also known as laver; kelp, also called kombu; wakame, hijiki, and arame (which are brown); and red dulse, which contains the highest iron concentration of any food source. Agar-agar, known as kanten in Japan, is used as a jelling or thickening agent, and Corsican seaweed is sold as a worming herb. Agar-agar and Corsican seaweed come with special instructions; the other sea vegetables listed here can be powdered and added to your pet's food.

N.R. Seaweed Mineral Food, developed by Juliette de Bairacli Levy, contains powdered seaweed, nettles, rosemary, comfrey, and cleavers. The label recommends a pinch per day for cats and small dogs, ⅛ to ¼ teaspoon per day for medium dogs, ¼ to ½ teaspoon per day for large dogs, and double these amounts for pigment, coat, or nutritional problems. To make similar powders, see pages 92 and 152–158.

Unrefined Sea Salt

One of the most important supplements for any pet is salt—not any salt, but unrefined, unprocessed sea salt, which contains only 80 to 83 percent sodium chloride. The remaining 17 to 20 percent consists of moisture and up to eighty-four trace elements in the proportions needed by all of the earth's animals.

Sprinkle a small amount of unrefined sea salt on fatty foods to improve digestion and assimilation. Add a pinch to each bowl of drinking water and to every meal, using more for large animals and less for small pets. A total of up to ½ teaspoon unrefined sea salt per 30 to 40 pounds of body weight every day or every other day is recommended.

Do not use refined table salt, kosher salt, or sea salt that has been boiled or heated during processing. If the salt is bright white or has the familiar taste of table salt, it won't contribute to your pet's good health. Look for naturally dried sea salt that is slightly gray in color, with a taste that's different from that of table salt.

For information on using unrefined sea salt to produce lactic acid fermented vegetables, see page 35.

When diarrhea causes dehydration and the loss of essential minerals, conventional veterinarians recommend electrolyte replacement products such as those sold for human infants, but their ingredients include refined salt, chemical preservatives, and artificial flavors. Gatorade and other sports drinks have similar formulas. It is easy to make your own superior product using the following recipe.

ELECTROLYTE REPLACEMENT FORMULA

Recommended for dogs or cats suffering from diarrhea, dehydration, heat stress, or physical exhaustion.

Combine 2 cups water, 1 tablespoon unrefined sea salt, ¼ teaspoon liquid colloidal trace minerals and ½ cup raw honey. If the cause of the problem is water contamination, use bottled water or boil filtered tap water. Let the animal drink freely or, if necessary, use a spoon or eyedropper to feed 1 tablespoon per 5 pounds of body weight every two to three hours.

Apple Cider Vinegar

Many herbalists recommend vinegar for pets because it can be poured over garlic and other herbs to make medicinal tinctures. Even without those herbs, cider vinegar can be an important ingredient in your pet's diet. Use any raw, unpasteurized, unheated, organic vinegar, such as Bragg Organic Apple Cider Vinegar, sold in health food stores. Apple cider is the most common vinegar, but raw, unpasteurized rice and wine vinegars are also available. Do not use a vinegar that is uniformly clear, such as the cider vinegar sold in supermarkets for pickle making, or most of the rice and wine vinegars sold in markets and health food stores. These are "dead" vinegars with none of the enzymes and other live factors that make raw, unpasteurized vinegar so valuable.

Long a folk remedy, cider vinegar has been shown to improve the health of dairy cows, horses, dogs, cats, and other animals. It reduces common infections, aids whelping, improves stamina, prevents muscle fatigue after exercise, increases resistance to disease, and protects against food poisoning. Cider vinegar normalizes acid levels in the stomach, improves digestion and the assimilation of nutrients, reduces intestinal gas and fecal odors, helps cure constipation, alleviates some of the symptoms of arthritis, and helps prevent bladder stones and urinary tract infections.

The only pets for whom vinegar is not recommended are those with a chronic yeast infection caused by organisms such as *Candida albicans* or those with an overly acidic system. Vinegar is believed to feed, reactivate, or exacerbate these conditions. However, animals fed a well-balanced raw diet and sufficient acidophilus to replenish the body's beneficial bacteria may be able to consume vinegar despite a history of candidiasis.

Add cider vinegar directly to food or drinking water, starting with small amounts and building up to ½ to 1 teaspoon per 15 pounds of body weight for dogs and cats (1 teaspoon per day for the average cat, 1 tablespoon for a 50-pound dog, or 2 tablespoons for a 90-pound dog). By gradually adding small doses to your pet's diet over time, you can help even the most finicky eater to accept this valuable food.

See page 145 for making herbal tinctures with raw vinegar; see page 168 for using cider vinegar externally as a flea and tick repellent.

Aloe Vera

The same succulent that offers relief from sunburn, insect bites and skin irritation has practical uses in pet care. The juice or gel of aloe vera, which is sold as a beverage, can be added to food to help prevent intestinal worms, improve the skin and coat, improve joint mobility, relieve arthritis symptoms, improve digestion, and help clear kidney, bladder, and urinary tract infections. When the leaf is cut open and applied externally, its inner gel speeds the healing of hot spots, skin conditions, burns, and wounds and has a cooling, soothing effect.

Aloe vera is easy to grow indoors in all climates and outdoors in mild weather. When moving aloe vera plants outdoors for the summer, place them where they will receive indirect light, not scorching sun. For best results, use plants at least three years old.

When adding the fresh leaf to food, peel it carefully to make sure that none of the bitter inner rind comes off with the gel; the rind and its yellow juice contain a powerful laxative. Aloe vera juice is sold in most health food stores, supermarkets and pharmacies. Because aloe vera has a slightly citrus or astringent taste, use it in small amounts until your pet grows accustomed to its flavor. Increase the dosage until you are giving up to 1 teaspoon of aloe vera gel or juice per 10 pounds of body weight daily as a general tonic (use half this amount if the product is concentrated) or up to 1 tablespoon per 10 pounds in the treatment of serious illnesses.

Quality is an important consideration for aloe vera shoppers, and labels can be difficult to decipher. Juices and gels labeled "cold processed" are actually pasteurized, and many contain chemical preservatives. Some are "whole leaf" preparations, which include the laxative outer rind, some contain only the inner gel, and some contain flavoring agents, artificial colors, sugar, high-fructose corn syrup, ascorbic acid (synthetic vitamin C), or other questionable ingredients. The most expensive products are powders containing isolated fractions of the plant, the most expensive juices and gels are sold by multilevel marketers, and dramatic advertising claims are common. Look for reputable manufacturers, organically grown aloe vera, and products free of artificial colors and flavoring agents.

Bee Pollen, Royal Jelly, and Bee Propolis

Some pet nutritionists think highly of bee products and some do not. Although she recommends honey in all of her pet books, Juliette de Bairacli Levy now asks her American lecture tour audiences not to use honey, royal jelly, bee pollen, or bee propolis because our bees are seriously stressed by environmental factors such as loss of habitat, exposure to pesticides, and infection by mites. If you can find a local beekeeper whose hives are healthy, your pets will enjoy and probably benefit from raw honey, especially honey in the comb, which can be added to food or given as a treat.

Bee pollen is a rich source of amino acids and vitamin B12, and it is widely reported to improve endurance, promote longevity, aid recovery from chronic illness, and help prevent disease. Many other foods and supplements have these same benefits. What makes bee pollen unique is that local pollen has helped many people and some dogs overcome summer allergies.

To use bee pollen for allergies, consider starting with very tiny doses, such as one grain of locally produced bee pollen on the tongue every day for a week, followed by two grains per day for a week, then three grains per day for a week. Some people are so allergic to bee pollen that half a teaspoon can send them into shock, and I suspect some dogs may have a similar reaction. If your dog shows no adverse reaction by the fourth week, try ⅛ teaspoon once per day, then as much as ¼ teaspoon per 25 pounds of body weight for a week or two. This strategy works best if begun in late winter or very early spring, well before local pollens are spread by the wind.

Flower pollen, which is collected by hand, does not contain the weed pollens commonly found in bee pollen, thus providing bee pollen's benefits without the threat of allergic reactions from ragweed and other problem plants. Flower pollen has been shown to be an effective treatment for prostate enlargement in men. It probably has the same effect in male dogs, and so might bee pollen.

Royal jelly is the substance nurse bees manufacture from pollen to feed the queen bee, who grows substantially larger and lives far longer than her sisters. This concentrated source of nutrients has been marketed as an immune system booster, antiaging compound, and virility drug. Some have used it to increase stamina and endurance in working dogs, to improve fertility in breeding dogs and cats, and to enhance the health of animals with nutritional deficiencies or wasting diseases. Pure royal jelly is one of the most expensive supplements on the market. Most royal jelly products combine royal jelly with raw honey.

Propolis is sometimes called "bee glue" because bees collect the sap of polar buds and the resin of coniferous trees, mix it with enzymes, beeswax, and pollen, and use it to repair cracks in the hive, coat larval cells, form protective openings that allow only bees to enter the hive, and

Need help finding a supplement or other product? See the Resources at the back of this book for recommended manufacturers and distributors.

embalm any rodent that might invade the hive. As a result, despite its warmth and humidity, the interior of a bee hive is more sterile than most hospitals.

Bee propolis is considered one of the strongest natural antibiotics and disinfectants known; it has antibacterial, antifungal, antimicrobial, antiseptic, and antiviral properties. Propolis is widely used to support the immune system and as a specific for cancer, urinary tract infections, throat swelling, open wounds, sinus congestion, bronchitis, gastritis, circulatory disorders, and virus infections such as colds and flu in people and corresponding illnesses in dogs and cats.

Some physicians and veterinarians believe propolis has a stimulating effect on the thymus gland. Research conducted in Eastern Europe and Austria indicates that propolis may repair cellular damage caused by X rays, kill cancer cells while leaving healthy cells intact, and rapidly heal stomach ulcers.

Wheat Grass, Rye Grass, and Other Cereal Grasses

Cereal grasses are nutritional powerhouses rich in chlorophyll, amino acids, minerals (especially potassium, calcium, and magnesium), vitamins, enzymes, and protein. They have a strong cleansing action and have been used for detoxification in pets and people, the correction of nutritional deficiencies, and the treatment of cancer, atopic dermatitis, pancreatitis, digestive problems, skin and coat conditions, insomnia, anemia, and respiratory diseases. Adding finely minced or chopped grass to a cat's food also helps prevent hair balls. All cereal grasses have a deodorizing effect, that improves the animal's breath and body odor.

Wheat, rye, oat, kamut, spelt, barley, and other grasses are easy to grow (see page 33), as is the "lettuce" of seeds such as buckwheat and sunflower. Barley grass is especially recommended because of its high B-vitamin content, but all grasses offer health benefits. Grow a variety, alternating grains from one week or month to the next. If your dog or cat is allergic to wheat, he may not be allergic to wheat grass and almost certainly will not have a problem tolerating barley grass, oat grass, rye grass, buckwheat lettuce, or sunflower lettuce. Buckwheat lettuce is a rich source of the bioflavonoid rutin and, with its red stems, makes a colorful addition to your own salads.

Cereal grass products, especially powders, are popular pet supplements. Powders are convenient, so if you aren't able to grow your own grasses, look for products that are grown organically and dried at low temperature. Wheat grass and barley grass from Pines International (see Resources) are grown under conditions that produce unusually high concentrations of vitamins and minerals.

Now that an Australian manufacturer has patented an extract of rye grass called Oralmat and tested it against asthma and other illnesses, this grass may rival wheat grass as an herbal cure-all for people and pets. Preliminary reports claim that very small quantities (3 drops under the tongue two or three times per day for adults and children) improve not only asthma but also allergies, colds, flu, diabetes, and infections caused by viruses, fungi, and bacteria. Placebo-controlled clinical trials are under way in Australia, with researchers reporting "extremely promising" preliminary results in the treatment of asthma. Rye grass is so easy to grow that giving your dog or cat a daily dose is both simple and inexpensive.

Because grasses are difficult for dogs and cats to digest, finely mince or grind wheat grass, rye grass, and other cereal grasses before serving. Add small amounts at first, then up to a teaspoon or more per 10 pounds of body weight every other day.

If you have a wheat grass juicer (centrifugal juicers won't work; you need a hydraulic press, screw press, or macerating juicer for this task), add tiny amounts of juice to your pet's food or water. Green juices are like vitamin/mineral/chlorophyll supplements. Start with just a few drops and gradually increase to about ¼ teaspoon per day for a 10-pound cat and 1 teaspoon per day for a 50-pound dog. Because wheat grass juice should be used soon after juicing, freeze leftover juice in ice cube trays, transfer the frozen cubes to heavy plastic bags for freezer storage, and thaw the cubes as needed.

Green juices are powerful medicines that should be used sparingly. Too much too fast can cause dizziness, vomiting, diarrhea, and other symptoms of rapid detoxification. Be sure your pet tolerates green juices well before increasing the amount you use.

Microalgae (Chlorella, Spirulina, Blue-Green Algae)

Billions of years ago, algae covered the oceans. The first photosynthesizing organisms on our planet, they are believed to have made the earth hospitable to future life by converting carbon dioxide to oxygen, thus creating our atmosphere. Spirulina, chlorella, and blue-green algae are among the world's most widespread herbs and in recent years have become quite popular. Nearly every line of pet supplements has at least two or three products containing microalgae. Not every strain is edible, but the species sold as food supplements are nontoxic and rich in chlorophyll, amino acids, vitamins, minerals, and protein.

Spirulina, named for its cell's spiral shape, is the only microalgae visible to the naked eye. Spirulina is popular among vegetarians, athletes, expectant mothers, senior citizens, and others who want to improve or maintain their health. First studied by scientists in the 1940s, spirulina was found to contain 65 to 70 percent protein, the eight essential amino acids, abundant vitamin B12, and other nutrients.

Chlorella, another ancient single-celled algae, derives its name from its high chlorophyll content. Chlorophyll repairs cells, increases hemoglobin in the blood, and speeds cell growth. In addition to being sold by itself, chlorella appears in many pet products that combine "green" ingredients, such as the other microalgae, wheat or barley grass juice, alfalfa, and green vegetables. Processing that breaks chlorella's cell wall is said to improve assimilation.

Blue-green algae, the popular name for a strain of *Aphanizaomenon*, grows on lakes and ponds. Like spirulina and chlorella, blue-green algae contains chlorophyll, vitamins, minerals, protein, amino acids, and other nutrients.

Are there significant differences between spirulina, chlorella, and blue-green algae, or between wild harvested and cultivated strains of each? According to researchers not affiliated with manufacturers, little is to be gained from comparing their individual merits. Nearly all descriptions of one type's superiority or another's inferiority come from manufacturers' promotional literature. Research conducted in Japan, Mexico, the United States, and other countries indicates that similar results can be expected from all three.

While spirulina and chlorella have long safety records, the blue-green algae harvested from Oregon's Klamath Lake is newer and less widely used. Occasional reports of dogs dying after drinking algae-contaminated water from Klamath Lake have appeared in dog magazines. In November 1996, *Vegetarian Times* reported that *Microcystis*, a toxic algae that can cause fatal liver damage, had been discovered in Klamath Lake. Owners considering the use of this supplement should look for updated safety reports from the manufacturers and in pet-related newsletters and magazines. As with any herbal supplement, consider using any algae product in courses, such as five days on and two days off for four to six weeks, then switch to a different microalgae.

Yeast and the Yeast Controversy

Brewer's yeast has become a controversial pet supplement in recent years because of the low-quality yeast used in many products. Veterinarian Alfred Plechner considers it a dangerous allergen, and Juliette de Bairacli Levy has denounced it for decades. Brewer's yeast was originally a waste product of beer brewing, and the brewer's yeast sold to pet food manufacturers was literally and figuratively the dregs of the process. A yeast residue might have been used and reused until it had no life left, at which time it was discarded and sold as animal feed.

Allergic reactions are common among animals fed a low-quality brewer's yeast. A high percentage of dogs with skin allergies have been shown to be yeast-sensitive. Another claim is that dogs cannot digest brewer's yeast.

At the same time, nutritional yeast and brewer's yeast are the foundation of many popular supplements, including those developed or endorsed by Richard Pitcairn, Anitra Frazier, Robert Goldstein, and others. Whenever researchers announce that brewer's yeast does not repel fleas, readers of health magazines write letters of protest, claiming the opposite.

The primary yeast cultivated by supplement manufacturers is *Saccharomyces cerevisiae*. Its nutritional content depends on the growth medium used to produce it, and its label name depends on the maker. For example, one manufacturer grows *S. cerevisiae* on hops and labels the product brewer's yeast; the same company grows *S. cerevisiae* on molasses and calls it nutritional yeast; a second company grows *S. cerevisiae* on sugar beets and calls it brewer's yeast. Some pet supplement makers claim that all brewer's yeast has a parasite-repelling high sulfur content and bitter taste unless the yeast has been debittered to make it more palatable. Neither of the brewer's yeasts described here is debittered, however, and both have a low sulfur content and sweet taste, while the nutritional yeast grown on molasses has a high sulfur content and bitter taste. If you are looking for yeast that will help repel fleas, compare the sulfur content of different brands.

Yeast has been shown to help animals resist infection. In a poultry study, *Saccharomyces boulardii*, the strain used to grow torulla yeast, was added to the feed of half the chickens being tested. All of the chickens were then orally inoculated with *Salmonella* bacteria. Only 5 percent of those fed the yeast developed salmonella colonies in their intestines, compared to 70 percent of the control group. Some owners feed their birds and other pets brewer's yeast, a close cousin of torulla, to help prevent the growth of undesirable bacteria.

Whatever its growth medium, premium quality brewer's or nutritional yeast was never used in beer brewing and is not a waste product. It is a rich source of B vitamins, amino acids, selenium, chromium, potassium, phosphorus, magnesium, copper, manganese, iron, zinc, and other trace elements.

As nutritious as it is, even the highest quality brewer's yeast can disrupt the life of an animal who is sensitive to yeast. If your dog or cat displays any allergic response to brewer's yeast, read labels carefully and avoid products that contain yeast of any type. After several weeks, if you would like to reintroduce yeast, try a high-quality liquid yeast (see Resources for this chapter) in small doses at widely spaced intervals and observe your pet's reaction.

Diatomaceous Earth

Diatomaceous earth is a powder made from fossilized, microscopic one-celled plants called diatoms. Deposits of diatoms, which are ground to create diatomaceous earth, cover large areas around the world. Two types of diatomaceous earth are sold in the United States, one used in swimming pool filters, the other an untreated "food grade" powder sold to gardeners as a slug and snail deterrent. A growing number of pet owners are adding the second type to their animals' dinners.

When diatoms were tested as a grain protectant, feeding tests were conducted on laboratory animals to determine toxicity. Researchers noticed that the animals fed diatoms were in better health than those fed a normal diet. In subsequent tests, young diatom-fed animals gained weight faster than control animals and had fewer problems with intestinal parasites. Diatoms remove existing worms and prevent reinfestation by scouring the intestines, irritating and damaging the parasites' soft bodies. When added to a cat's food, diatomaceous earth helps prevent hair balls.

Although diatomaceous earth is considered a safe addition to live-stock grain and other dry foods, keep in mind recent warnings of lung damage caused by inhaling this powder. Diatomaceous earth works because of its sharp edges, which cut soft tissue and kill flea larvae, garden slugs, and other soft-bodied animals. This product should be handled carefully and gently stirred into wet food until damp. The recommended amount is ½ teaspoon per 10 pounds of body weight.

Willard Water (Catalyst Altered Water)

Willard Water, also called catalyst altered water, is a concentrate sold in some health food stores and by mail (see Resources). John Willard, Ph.D., a professor of chemistry, developed this substance while working in oil fields. After much experimentation, he patented two forms of the concentrate. Willard Water is sold as a clear or dark concentrate for mixing with "good" water, *good* being defined as uncontaminated spring water, distilled water, or filtered tap water. The treated water, which reduces stress and improves digestion and the assimilation of nutrients in humans and animals, was the subject of a 1980 *60 Minutes* television program and two subsequent books.

I was interested in Willard Water's ability to destroy chlorine and act as a preservative and disinfectant, so in 1991, the year he died, I corresponded with Dr. Willard. He said, "In answer to your question, I will give you some information that is not public knowledge. Take one-third of an ounce (10 c.c.) of clear Willard Water extract in one gallon of good water (use distilled or deionized water if you're not sure). Put the dilute solution in a mist sprayer and spray it on hair, wounds, food, raw meat, etc., to disinfect. It reacts with the air to become a powerful oxidizing agent and preservative. I have cleaned up two hospitals with very hazardous contamination. Why the micelle operates as it does is known only to God. We scientists have never found anything else with such properties. In answer to your question regarding its use with raw milk or fresh juice, add one ounce of either clear or dark Willard Water per gallon, or one and one-half teaspoons per quart. We discovered this with an old Swiss cheesemaker. Milk tastes richer and keeps fresh longer."

I always add a pinch of unrefined sea salt and a splash of Willard Water concentrate to drinking water and to fresh, raw juice for all of us, pets as well as people. Willard Water has been used and tested on animals for decades, and the result is a long list of documented improvements with no adverse side effects. The most frequently reported claims from farmers, veterinarians, breeders, trainers, handlers, and pet owners are improved digestion, calmness, improved coat luster and eye sparkle, improved gait, resistance to stress-related illness, increased immunity, and fewer fights among dogs. Willard reported that when animals with infections were treated with antibiotics, veterinarians were able to reduce the drug dosage by half or more if the micelle was administered at the same time.

For pets under stress or during hot weather, Willard suggested adding 1 tablespoon to each quart of drinking water, which is twice the usual concentration and which is appropriate for animals undergoing treatment for cancer. Otherwise, use 2 tablespoons per gallon for daily use or a more economical dose of 1 teaspoon per gallon. Even in extremely dilute solutions, the extract has improved the health of farm animals and domestic pets. The only potential side effect when animals drink more than they need is mild diarrhea.

Externally, it can be sprayed or applied to cuts, wounds, burns, eye infections, cataracts, poison ivy rashes, and other injuries to speed healing. Added to pet shampoo or rinse water, it softens rough coats and makes fur more manageable. My most dramatic demonstration of this was a test I conducted on an old wool sweater after I read John Willard's assertion that adding his concentrate to wash water prevents wool from shrinking. Skeptical, I set the machine to a gentle cycle and added hot water, 1 tablespoon Willard Water concentrate, and regular laundry detergent. The sweater, which didn't shrink, looks newer and fluffier than it has in years.

Methyl-Sulfonyl-Methane (MSM)

In the rapidly growing world of nutritional supplements, one of the most popular is methyl-sulfonyl-methane (MSM), a form of sulfur found in plants, fruits, vegetables, meat, and garden soil. Sulfur is essential to the formation of blood proteins, amino acids, connective tissue, and healthy skin. It activates the utilization of thiamine, vitamin C, biotin, and pantothenic acid, maintains the body's pH balance (acid/alkaline), and participates in the manufacture of bile and insulin.

Plant-derived sulfur is in short supply in America because of depleted farm soils and because the heat of cooking or processing destroys it. Since its development as a food supplement, MSM has been shown to help prevent food allergies and sensitivities, relieve heartburn and other digestive problems, improve arthritis symptoms, relieve muscle pain, improve lung function, eliminate parasites, and possibly prevent cancer.

Dogs and cats on a well-balanced diet of fresh, raw foods receive natural MSM in every meal, but supplemental MSM may be helpful in the treatment of allergies, joint pain, gastrointestinal problems, low energy, muscle injuries, respiratory infections, or parasites, especially in animals that have been regularly fed commercial pet food. Holistic veterinarians often prescribe MSM powder at the rate of 50 to 100 grams per 10 pounds of body weight mixed with food. Also recommended are MSM eyedrops for eye infections, injuries, glaucoma, cataracts, and ear cleansing (this is a multipurpose product), MSM shampoo for improved skin and coat, and MSM powder mixed with aloe vera gel or water for tooth and gum treatment (apply on a toothbrush or gauze wipe).

Although its promoters claim that this supplement has no adverse side effects, MSM may contribute to nutritional imbalances. In his *Nutrition & Healing* newsletter, Jonathan Wright, M.D., warns that MSM can strip the body of the trace element molybdenum. He recommends supplemental molybdenum for those taking MSM in large doses or for long periods. MSM is probably most helpful to dogs and cats that have been on commercial pet food, but it is not a substitute for a natural diet.

Seacure

Seacure is a nutritional supplement made from deep-sea fish that are predigested by a fermentation process developed in Uruguay. The powder is rich in amino acids and peptides, easily assimilated, and hypoallergenic. Unlike synthetic amino acids, Seacure is a whole-food supplement. In addition to protein, it contains unsaturated fats and mineral ash, including calcium and phosphorus. Seacure is recommended for a variety of conditions in people and pets of all ages, for its use speeds wound healing, boosts immunity, improves digestion, and relieves joint pain. In extensive tests on premature, underweight, malnourished human infants who were given 1 to 2 grams daily, the babies' weight, digestion, and immune functions improved dramatically, and in many, allergies disappeared.

Pet owners and veterinarians have reported improvements in immune function, joint flexibility, digestion, allergies, wound healing, stamina, and behavior after adding Seacure, which has a pleasant (if you're a dog or cat) fishy smell, to their animals' food. Seacure can be an important aid to detoxification, as its amino acids provide essential nutrients for the liver (see page 96).

Colostrum and Lactoferrin

Colostrum is the first milk a mammal produces after giving birth. In dogs, cats, cows, and humans, this milk is so rich in immune system support that it protects newborns from infections and intestinal disorders. Colostrum affects thirty-two growth factors including muscle, cartilage, connective tissue, body weight, and lean muscle.

Colostrum and lactoferrin protect the mucous membrane, interfere with the reproduction of harmful bacteria, activate T-cells which attack invading organisms, repair damaged muscle and cartilage tissue, and improve muscle tone. They are recommended for any animal that is weak, elderly, susceptible to illness, or fighting or recovering from any disease.

Derived from cow's milk, colostrum supplements are reported to enhance immune function in dogs, cats, humans, and other animals. Lactoferrin, one of the immune factors in colostrum, is also sold as an immune-enhancing supplement. For information regarding these products and their production, consult individual manufacturers.

Beta 1, 3 D Glucan

Supplements that claim to enhance the immune system have become a very big business, and it is difficult to separate advertising hype from documented results. One supplement that has performed well in clinical trials conducted at Harvard Medical School and other institutions is Beta 1, 3 D Glucan, a naturally occurring compound derived from the cell wall of baker's yeast (*Saccharomyces cerevisiac*). Sold under the brand name Immutol (see Resources), this substance has been shown to promote rapid wound healing, reduce cholesterol levels, protect against damage by radiation, and inhibit tumor growth. In addition, it has been used to treat allergies, herpes, bacterial and viral infections, bronchitis, internal parasites, systemic yeast infections, periodontal or gum disease, pneumonia, diabetes, environmental illness, arthritis, and other illnesses without adverse side effects.

Make-Your-Own Supplement Blends

Combining supplement ingredients ahead of time simplifies meal preparation. If you plan to add several powders or supplemental foods to your pet's dinner every night, consider mixing them into blends that can be given daily or on alternating days. If you grow wheat grass, sprout grain, and prepare lactic acid fermented vegetables, your refrigerated mixture of enzyme-rich "live foods" will last for several days. Below are three examples of do-it-yourself blends. Substitute, add, and adjust ingredients as desired.

Medicinal herbs, described in the following chapter, and commercial products such as Seacure and powdered colostrum, can be added to supplement blends as needed. To make a one-week supply of any blend, mix together the week's total amount of each supplement powder. To determine the correct amount to feed, add the recommended daily amounts of all ingredients and label the container accordingly.

When adding a supplement powder to your pet's food, soak the meat in hot water to warm it. Drain the meat but leave it wet. Sprinkle the powder over the meat and stir until it is completely damp. If necessary, add more water, a splash of aloe vera juice, or other liquids.

CAROB BLEND

Recommended for dogs of all ages for improved skin and coat, resistance to internal parasites, and overall good health.

Combine 1 cup carob powder, 1 cup diatomaceous earth, 3 tablespoons powdered chlorella, 2 tablespoons powdered wheat grass juice, 5 teaspoons unrefined sea salt, and 4 teaspoons powdered kelp. Double or triple these ingredients for large or giant breeds. Handle the diatomaceous earth with care (see page 87) to avoid inhaling it. Combine ingredients in a glass jar and shake or invert to mix well.

Add approximately 1 teaspoon per 5 pounds of body weight to food every day for two weeks or every other day for a month. Conversions: 1 tablespoon for a 15-pound dog, 2 tablespoons for a 30-pound dog, 4 tablespoons (¼ cup) for a 60-pound dog, 8 tablespoons (½ cup) for a 120-pound dog, and so forth.

The carob in this blend appeals to most dogs because it tastes like chocolate, a favorite (but forbidden) flavor. Although most carob powder is roasted, the Resources lists sources of raw carob powder. This blend provides essential vitamins, minerals, enzymes, and other nutrients, and the diatomaceous earth helps repel worms.

KELP BLEND

Recommended for all dogs and cats for good health, correct pigment, immune system support, and glandular health.

Combine 1 part unrefined sea salt, 2 parts powdered kelp, and 2 parts powdered wheat grass or barley grass juice. Add approximately ⅛ teaspoon per 5 pounds of body weight to food per day. For protection from internal parasites and to help prevent hair balls, measure the combined blend and add an equal amount of diatomaceous earth (see page 86). Add approximately ¼ teaspoon of this second blend per 5 pounds of body weight per day.

Because kelp has a faintly fishy odor that most cats and dogs enjoy, this nutritious blend is easy to use. If your cat doesn't like it, try adding tuna powder for flavor (see Resources), or mix it with your pet's favorite odoriferous food.

SPROUTED GRAIN/VEGETABLE BLEND FOR CATS AND DOGS

Recommended for all dogs and cats as a source of vitamins, enzymes, and minerals.

Sprout whole wheat, rye, or other grain as described on pages 29–30. Prepare lactic acid fermented vegetables such as carrots and cucumbers as described on page 35, handling them with a slotted spoon or partially draining before using. Combine approximately 1 cup of each in a food processor or blender and puree until the sprouting grain is pulverized. Add 1 or 2 cloves of raw garlic and, if available, a handful of freshly cut wheat grass or other grass, cutting it into small pieces with scissors as you add it to the mixture. Puree until all ingredients are well combined. If desired, add as a natural preservative 2 or 3 tablets of food-source vitamin C (or, if you must use a synthetic vitamin C, calcium ascorbate with bioflavonoids) plus 2 or 3 capsules or tablets of natural vitamin E. Refrigerate.

Consider this blend to be the contents of a prey animal's stomach. Feed small amounts to cats and larger amounts to dogs, keeping in mind the prey animal model. A cat dining on one or two mice would consume less than a teaspoon of partly digested grain. A dog dining on a wild hare or chicken might consume only a tablespoon or two of partly digested grass, grain, and vegetable matter. Canines in the wild dine on small animals such as hares and birds far more often than they dine on large game.

Because dogs and cats in the wild occasionally find prey with full stomachs, a larger-than-average serving once a week or so is in keeping with the prey animal model. Samantha, who weighs 60 pounds, receives 1 rounded tablespoon of this blend Monday through Friday, and our cats Pepper and Pumpkin receive ½ teaspoon each. On Saturday, Pepper and Pumpkin receive a rounded tablespoon each, and Samantha eats whatever is left, usually ½ to 1 cup. Sunday is our fast day, with all of the animals receiving water only. On Monday I prepare a new mixture with a different sprouted grain, different pressed vegetables, and a different cereal grass or combination of salad greens, dandelion greens, and other fresh herbs.

Because its active enzymes will continue to work, this is a perishable mixture. Even freezing will not inactivate the enzymes, although cold temperatures slow their action. For freezer storage, spread the blend in an ice cube tray, then transfer frozen cubes to an airtight freezer bag. For best results, use the refrigerated blend within one week and use frozen servings within one month.

Detoxification

One of the most important functions herbs and nutritional supplements provide is support during detoxification. The detoxification process is ongoing in pets and people as the body breaks down and removes waste products. Old cells, cell waste products, unneeded hormones, the by-products of digestion, chemical residues, the waste products of internal parasites, the bodies of dead parasites, and other debris travel through the blood and lymph to the liver and kidneys, which filter them for removal in the urine and feces. Toxins that the body isn't able to eliminate quickly are stored in the liver or in body fat for later processing.

If you have ever gone without food for a day or two, overindulged in alcohol, consumed too much coffee, or abruptly changed your diet, you will recognize the symptoms of rapid detoxification. In addition to having headaches, fatigue, and diarrhea, you probably felt clammy, your skin and breath smelled awful, and you may have vomited. Dandruff, skin eruptions, bumps, rashes, and itching are additional symptoms.

Dogs and cats experience something similar when they go without food for a day or more, recover from illness, or adjust to a rapid change of diet. As with humans, the severity of symptoms depends on how much waste material is released for elimination and how well the body's filtering systems are working.

Pet owners must understand the mechanics of detoxification in order to prevent health problems that commonly result when we give supplements that stimulate this process, switch from commercial food to a raw diet, encourage pets to lose weight (losing fat releases toxins stored in fat), or fail to recognize symptoms of detoxification in animals that are under stress, are ill, or recovering from an illness.

For effective processing of waste products, the body needs key nutrients, including vitamins, minerals, and amino acids. If they aren't available or aren't provided in sufficient quantity, the system can be overwhelmed, resulting in rapid detoxification. The body actually can be poisoned, resulting in damage to the liver, kidney, heart, muscles, nerves, or brain, and even death. Animals at greatest risk are those that have been fed a commercial diet or a lifetime of home-prepared cooked food, exposed to chemical or environmental pollutants, treated with flea-killing insecticides, and dosed with pharmaceutical drugs such as antibiotics, heartworm medication, and systemic flea preventives.

Phase 1

During the first stage of elimination, the body identifies and separates waste products, toxins, and anything else that it doesn't need from the blood and lymph. Water-soluble material that can be excreted goes to the kidneys. Dehydration complicates the detoxification process, which is why all pets should have free access to clean drinking water and why pets that are recovering from illness, experiencing weight loss, changing to a natural diet, or eliminating intestinal parasites, or that have been treated with conventional drugs, should be given extra water in their food or encouraged to drink extra water throughout the day.

Everything that isn't water soluble and sufficiently small to be excreted in the animal's urine is sent to the liver. In the liver, substances are processed in two phases. In phase 1, waste products are made water soluble and sent to the kidneys for elimination. The liver uses antioxidants and key minerals such as vitamins A, C, and E, bioflavonoids, selenium, copper, superoxide dismutase (SOD), zinc, and manganese during this phase.

Phase 2

Anything that cannot be made water soluble in phase 1 goes to phase 2. "If a substance can't flow into the urine," wrote Nancy Scanlan, D.V.M., in the January 1996 *Natural Pet*, "it is usually more toxic than it started out. The original toxins become half-processed supertoxins." In phase 2, these supertoxins are attached to molecules such as amino acids and eliminated through the urine or intestines. During this phase, the liver uses glucuronic acid, sulfates from glutathione, acetyl-cysteine, and the amino acids taurine, arginine, ornithine, glutamine, and cysteine. In dogs and most other animals, but not in cats, the amino acid glycine is also needed.

When an animal is deficient in either phase 1 or phase 2 nutrients, backups and spillovers occur. Supertoxins traveling through the bloodstream searching for a home may find one in fatty tissue, or they may stay in the blood, infecting healthy tissue and causing new illnesses. Holistic health practitioners often observe that taking large amounts of antioxidant supplements can cause fatigue and other unpleasant symptoms, suggesting that the patient is stimulating phase 1 detoxification without providing the amino acids required by the liver for phase 2. In dogs and cats as well as people, insufficient quantities of either family of nutrients can be deleterious.

Mitochondria are energy production units in the cells, and they are several times more sensitive to the presence of toxins and the lack of key nutrients than are normal cells. Mitochondria need vitamins E, K, and B-complex, niacin, coenzyme Q10, and the amino acid carnitine. A lack of nutritional support for mitochondria contributes to the overwhelming fatigue associated with rapid detoxification.

According to Scanlan, it is impossible to predict if and when an animal will be so stressed by detoxification that its life is in danger. Normal laboratory tests, such as liver enzyme tests and kidney function tests, can show only that an organ has been damaged, not whether it is in the early stages of illness. In addition, she noted, pet owners sometimes contribute to "toxic detox" by providing the antioxidant supplements that stimulate phase 1 while neglecting the amino acids needed for phase 2. Both types of nutrients are required in sufficient quantities to keep partially processed toxins from circulating throughout the body.

To Fast or Not to Fast

The feeding cycle modeled after Mother Nature, in which dogs and cats are given only water one day per week, may be too stressful for some animals. If your pet is more than five years old; has been fed a commercial or home-cooked diet; has been seriously ill or under stress; was at any time exposed to chemical pesticides, dosed with prescription heartworm medication, or given systemic flea preventives or other drugs; is losing weight or has an unusually rapid metabolism, do not give a water-only fast one day per week. Instead, let the digestive system rest by feeding light foods such as carrot juice for a dog, a soupy puree of meat or organically raised chicken liver and water for a cat, or raw goat's milk with lactase and acidophilus for either. Supplement this liquid fare with antioxidants for phase 1 detoxification and Seacure (see page 90) or other amino acid blends for phase 2.

For healthy pets on a well-balanced raw diet, the nutrients needed for efficient detoxification are provided in abundance, and supplementation can be confined to fast days. For example, kelp, cod liver oil, and a food-source multiple vitamin/mineral supplement provide abundant phase 1 and phase 2 nutrients. During detoxification, synthetic vitamins are a cause of stress, and for pets on a bone-based raw diet, single-mineral supplements are unnecessary and potentially damaging. Liver itself contains most of the nutrients the liver needs, as described on page 22, and various herbs help the detoxification process, as described on pages 203–208.

Whether you are adopting a more natural feeding schedule or considering a fast for therapeutic purposes, it is important to understand the process of detoxification and to provide the nutrients your pet needs for safe, effective elimination.

Chapter 3

Your Pet's Herbal Pharmacy

B y far, the world's most widely used natural therapy is herbal medicine. Every culture on every continent has experimented with local plants and developed a tradition of diagnosis and use, a repertoire based on experience and observation.

My teacher Rosemary Gladstar offers sensible advice to those who are new to these traditions. "In order for herbs to be effective," she says, "they must be used with consistency. This is probably the most difficult aspect of herbalism for people in the twentieth century. In our age of quick fixes and instant medicine, the old art of brewing and using herbal tea seems antiquated and time-consuming." On the contrary, she explains, it's really easy and practical. So is the use of herbal powders, capsules, tinctures, extracts, oils, salves, essential oils, and other products.

The real advantage of medicinal herbs, especially for pet owners," explains Gladstar, "is that they work both gently and thoroughly. Herbs don't have the side effects of pharmaceutical drugs, but they are powerful medicines nonetheless. Our pets are usually closer to Mother Nature than we are, and they have a special affinity for her remedies."

Deb Soule, owner of Avena Botanicals Herbal Apothecary and an expert on herbal pet care, agrees. "The information the public receives about herbal medicine is often trendy and superficial," she says. "Because our culture is so accustomed to the methods of allopathic medicine, it is easy to look at herbs as simple replacements for pharmaceutical drugs, but this is a mistake. Herbs don't suppress symptoms the way drugs do; they go deeper, to the source of a health problem, and they are usually gentler and slower acting. When you use whole plant ingredients like blossoms, leaves, and roots, you're using versatile materials that don't have to be measured like prescription drugs. Your pets will respond to these gentle, effective remedies and live longer, healthier, happier lives."

Herbal First Aid for Your Pet

The following conditions can be quickly and successfully healed through the proper use of herbs. For best results and future good health, the herbal treatment should be accompanied by fresh, raw food (as described in chapter 1), daily exposure to natural light, pure water, clean air, regular exercise, and a peaceful environment. Refer to the pages indicated below for a suggested herbal therapy. These conditions and others are described in more detail in *The Encyclopedia of Natural Pet Care*.

Condition	Page Number
Abscesses and boils	163, 185, 190
Allergies	154, 162
Anemia	113
Anal glands, impacted	163
Anxiety	160, 180, 185
Arthritis	138, 154, 158, 181
Bad breath	154, 189
Bleeding, internal	140, 161

Condition	Page Number

On the Safety of Herbs

To say that herbs are controversial is an understatement. Cautions about their potential toxicity abound, and the U.S. Food and Drug Administration (FDA) is quick to issue warnings. Is the user really in danger?

In a few cases, yes. Foxglove, the source of digitalis, is a poisonous plant, as is belladonna (deadly nightshade). Some products manufactured in the United States have been recalled after users became ill from incorrectly identified imported herbs, including a European foxglove that was misidentified as plantain. A number of herbal products imported from China and Taiwan are contaminated with pharmaceutical drugs and other questionable ingredients. Responsible herbalists guard against accidental or intentional adulteration by growing or collecting the herbs they use, buying from reputable sources, and testing herbs purchased in bulk for their quality, purity, and identification.

At the same time, an herb can be 100 percent natural, correctly identified, organically grown, correctly processed, and still pose a hazard to you or your pet.

Ethnobotanist David Winston borrows a description from Native American medicine to introduce the wide range of properties herbs possess. "In the Cherokee tradition, there are three types of herbs," he explains. "There are food herbs, which can be used in large quantities and are very unlikely to create any type of adverse reaction. There are medicines that require more knowledge and should be used for specific conditions for a specified period of time because they are stronger and have the potential to cause adverse reactions if used incorrectly. Then there are poisons, which can cause serious adverse reactions up to and including death. This last group of herbs should be used only by people trained in their safe use and administered in very small doses."

Category 1: Safe "Food" Herbs

Dandelion, stinging nettle, chamomile, burdock root, calendula, lavender, echinacea, ginseng, raspberry leaf, parsley, and rosemary are examples of food herbs that have a long history of safe, effective use with pets. Many herbs with a more medicinal reputation belong to this category, too, such as hawthorn berry, which usually is classified as a heart medicine, saw palmetto berry, which prevents prostate enlargement, and valerian, a relaxing nervine. Also included are herbs described as tonics (which gradually restore and strengthen the entire system), alteratives (which gradually cleanse the blood), and adaptogens (which gradually restore balance throughout the body), all of which work best when taken daily for months or years. Most of the herbs mentioned in this book belong to category 1.

Category 2: Powerful Medicines

As more serious medicines, cascara sagrada and senna leaf are examples of the second category. These laxative herbs should be used in small doses and for a limited time to avoid bowel irritation, diarrhea, dehydration, and mineral imbalances. Other examples are the stimulant herb ma huang (ephedra), which should not be used by people with high blood pressure and is seldom recommended for pets, and herbs that contain caffeine, such as green tea, guarana, and kola nut. Large doses of the catalyst herb lobelia, which is both a nerve tonic and respiratory aid, can cause vomiting; large doses of the relaxing herb kava kava can interfere with coordination; and arnica, which in small doses is a specific for internal injuries, may cause heart problems and other complications in large doses.

Category 3: Toxic Herbs

Herbs from this category, such as the previously mentioned foxglove and belladonna, are true poisons. These herbs can be powerful medicines in minuscule doses but are not appropriate for home use.

Category 4: Topical Irritants

Some common herbs cause skin irritation and must be handled with care. Fresh rue rubbed on the skin as an insect repellent can cause a terrible rash. Rue repels insects when used as a companion plant in the garden and is an important ingredient in herbal supplements for dogs and cats, but it has never been recommended for use on human skin. Another insect-repelling plant is tansy, which, although less irritating than rue, affects some people adversely. A longhaired dog or cat might not break out in a rash, but someone stroking her fur might, so these herbs are not recommended for external application.

Herbs and Pregnancy

Most herb books contain a separate list of herbs to avoid during pregnancy. Although some of these lists are exceedingly cautious, it makes sense to avoid therapeutic doses of medicinal herbs during breeding, pregnancy, whelping, or nursing unless they are recommended for use at that time or are so nontoxic that they don't pose a threat. In general, small doses of therapeutic herbs are probably safe. For example, Juliette de Bairacli Levy's N.R. Herbal Antiseptic Tablets, which contain small amounts of wormwood, have been used on pregnant animals for half a century with no adverse effects. The larger wormwood quantities used in Hulda Clark's antiparasite program are not recommended, however. Angelica, black cohosh, blue cohosh, motherwort, and yarrow are known to stimulate uterine contractions. Many herbs that are safe in their natural state are far more likely to cause problems when concentrated as essential oils. Where developing kittens and puppies are concerned, it is better to err on the side of caution.

A number of books warn that aloe vera should not be used during breeding or the first trimester of pregnancy. These cautions, however, are based on the effects of evaporated and processed *Aloe ferox* (Cape aloe from South Africa) and *Aloe vulgaris* (the common aloe of North Africa and Southern Europe), which are concentrated laxatives with abortifacient properties. The juice or gel of aloe vera, an entirely different plant, does not cause uterine contractions and does not interfere with breeding, pregnancy, whelping, or nursing.

Scientific research sometimes adds to the confusion. In March 1999, researchers at Loma Linda University School of Medicine in Loma Linda, California, made headlines when they reported that four best-selling herbs might cause pregnancy risks. Hamster eggs and human sperm exposed to dilute solutions of St. John's wort, *Echinacea purpurea,* and *Ginkgo biloba* suffered damage, including a reduced ability of sperm to penetrate an egg, changes to the genetic material in sperm, poor sperm viability, and in the case of St. John's wort, mutation of a tumor suppressor gene. Of the herbs tested, only saw palmetto, which is commonly taken by men to relieve the symptoms of an enlarged prostate, did not damage eggs or sperm in the doses tested, though it did reduce the viability of sperm exposed to the herbal preparation for seven days.

The researchers noted that there is no evidence suggesting that people taking the recommended dosages of these herbs are adversely affected, for no data exist on the concentrations of these herbs in semen or blood serum, and the herbal doses tested may not represent amounts that actually reach eggs or sperm in people taking them. The same is true for dogs and cats. I wonder what results the researchers would have obtained if they had tested the effects of city tap water, cola beverages, aspirin, chemical preservatives, and artificial flavors on eggs and sperm.

Practicing herbalists, midwives, and breeders who have studied medicinal herbs are your best sources of information regarding the safe use of herbs during pregnancy.

The Problem with "Dangerous Plant" Lists

As a result of the explosion of interest in natural remedies, America's newspapers, magazines, and television news programs have interviewed experts of every description regarding the effectiveness, use, and safety of herbs. Because medicinal herbs are unfamiliar to most physicians, veterinarians, pharmacists, health care professionals, and scientists in the United States, these authorities often repeat inaccurate or incomplete information. In some cases, an herb is labeled dangerous because its berries are poisonous, because of a single documented allergic reaction, or because animals ingesting large amounts suffered adverse side effects.

It is always disconcerting to see dangerous category 3 plants such as aconite, deadly nightshade, foxglove, hemlock, jimsonweed, mayapple, and pokeweed listed as though health food stores sell their dried leaves for tea brewing, but some physicians who truly don't know the difference between safe and toxic herbs warn their patients away from *all* medicinal herbs simply because a few are dangerous. Others, with nothing but previously published warning lists to guide them, pass on information that was never accurate or has been since disproven. Some misrepresented herbs are especially helpful to dogs and cats. The following are a few examples.

Aloe vera. Although the wide use of this popular herb has made health-conscious Americans aware of its benefits for pets and people, it is sometimes listed as unsafe for internal consumption because the bitter juice of its inner rind has a laxative effect. Most bottled aloe vera juice or gel contains little or none of this ingredient. To use home-grown aloe vera, carefully pare the rind and rinse away any yellow or orange sap before adding the gel to your pet's food. When applying it to the skin, slice the leaf diagonally or vertically to expose the greatest amount of gel so that a licking dog or grooming cat will not swallow the sap. Aloe vera is a category 1 herb.

Arnica. An important first-aid item, arnica tincture is best known for its dramatic effect on bruises—and for its "external use only" labels. European physicians have long prescribed arnica tea or tincture as a cardiac agent, but it is such a powerful heart stimulant that it can be dangerous. In her popular book *Herbal Medicine*, Dian Dincin Buchman echoed many American herbalists when she wrote, "I must warn you that arnica is never to be used on open flesh wounds externally. Arnica may only be used on unbroken skin!"

But by taking such a cautious approach, say some experts, users deprive themselves of arnica's most important potential. In small doses, arnica can stop internal bleeding and stimulate healing, especially after trauma injuries. For emergency use, give 1 drop of arnica tincture, diluted in water, per 15 pounds of body weight two to four times daily. For cats and small dogs, use 1 drop twice a day.

This simple therapy saved the life of Rosie, a young tabby cat whose story appeared in the September 1983 *Tiger Tribe*. Rosie's encounter with a taxi resulted in a broken sacrum and broken tail. Because they believed she would never urinate or defecate normally, veterinarians recommended putting her to sleep. After a week of taking Herb Pharm's arnica drops twice per day, Rosie was eliminating normally and made a rapid recovery.

Ed Smith, the founder of Herb Pharm, told me that Rosie's story is typical, for arnica is a specific for injury-caused incontinence in people as

well as pets. A highly regarded herbalist and researcher, Smith finds no justification for the warnings on arnica products. In addition to its internal
use, he recommends applying it to bleeding wounds and other injuries to
reduce swelling, pain, and bruising.

Arnica is a category 2 herb that should be used with respect, but its
potential benefits far outweigh its risks. *Note:* Be sure your arnica tincture
is made with grain alcohol, not isopropyl (rubbing alcohol) or denatured
alcohol. If in doubt, contact the manufacturer.

Burdock root. This common Japanese vegetable is found in sushi bars,
health food stores, Japanese markets, and many herbal formulas. Reports
of its toxicity stem from a single instance in which a batch of burdock was
contaminated with belladonna root, which contains three toxic alkaloids,
including atropine. Some medical authorities continue to list burdock as
toxic. Burdock is a category 1 herb.

Castor oil. The ornate castor plant, a popular garden accent, can cause
allergic reactions, and its elaborately patterned seeds are so poisonous
that a single one can kill a dog or small child. The castor oil sold for pharmaceutical purposes has been treated to remove the seed's toxins. Castor
oil usually is applied externally, but when taken internally, it is a purgative
laxative. It is recommended by some pet care experts when an animal
becomes infected with a contagious illness or swallows something potentially harmful. Long-term internal use of castor oil is never recommended.

Chamomile. Chamomile is often blamed for allergic reactions, especially
in people who have ragweed allergies. In the past hundred years, only five
cases of chamomile allergy have been reported in the medical literature,
and some research suggests that chamomile actually helps alleviate allergic reactions such as hay fever. Chamomile is an exceptionally safe category 1 herb for pets and has important digestive, anti-inflammatory, and
relaxing benefits.

Chaparral. Chaparral received unfavorable publicity when it was blamed by the FDA for acute toxic hepatitis and a voluntary ban was initiated by sellers. Subsequent research failed to establish any connection between chaparral and the disease, so the herb is again available. Chaparral is important for pets. When added to food, it repels and helps eliminate worms and other parasites. As a tea, it can be applied to wounds and itching skin to speed healing. Chaparral kills most viruses, including the herpes virus, which can infect pregnant dogs and their puppies, and it has potent cancer-fighting properties. Despite its safety and effectiveness, chaparral continues to appear on "dangerous herb" lists. While most herbalists suggest using herbs other than chaparral for pets with liver disease, it is an excellent category 1 herb for all other canines and felines. See the Resources for Larreastat, a chaparral extract from which the plant's controversial oxidative components have been removed.

Coltsfoot. In 1987, a Swiss infant born with a severely damaged liver died. Every day of her pregnancy, the mother drank an expectorant tea containing coltsfoot. The tea contained senecionine, a pyrrolizidine alkaloid (PA), but its source was uncertain; it may not have been coltsfoot. As a precaution, the German government placed a one-year moratorium on the sale of coltsfoot. No other cases of potential coltsfoot toxicity were discovered and the ban was repealed. Coltsfoot preparations, including tinctures, teas, and syrups, are effective in treating respiratory illnesses in dogs and cats, including coughs, bronchitis, and other lung conditions. Despite its proven safety, coltsfoot is often listed as a dangerous herb that causes liver damage. It is instead a category 1 herb.

Comfrey. Comfrey has been removed from many pet supplements because it contains a class of compounds that, when isolated and fed in large doses, can cause liver damage and cancer in rats. In hundreds of years of use, no cases of human problems with comfrey have ever been documented, but in 1984 a woman who had been taking comfrey-pepsin tablets developed liver toxicity. Since then, three additional cases of human liver disease have been reported in people who took the herb.

The potentially harmful ingredients in comfrey are its PAs. Because of the plant's long history of safe use, many herbalists and pet owners continue to use it on a regular basis. Chopped, fresh comfrey, dried comfrey in capsules, or comfrey tinctures are given for improved digestion, skin and coat conditions, and the rapid healing of broken bones. Comfrey is a key ingredient in Juliette de Bairacli Levy's N.R. Seaweed Mineral Food, used by pets around the world, including pregnant animals, for more than fifty years with no adverse effects. It is also a key ingredient in the bone-repair tincture described on page 150, which has stimulated the reformation of bone in dogs with bone cancer.

Veterinarian Beverly Cappel cautions that she has seen dogs who began vomiting after taking several comfrey capsules daily for three to five weeks. When she tested the blood of these dogs, Cappel found elevated liver counts. She therefore recommends giving comfrey in food with caution, if at all. Whenever I tell this story to practicing herbalists, they suspect that the herb really wasn't comfrey, that the product was adulterated, or that the liver dysfunction was caused by something unrelated to comfrey.

Ed Smith isn't so sure. "Your comfrey might have no alkaloids at all," he told me, "or it might contain high concentrations. It all depends on the species, its growing conditions, and other unpredictable factors. You can't be sure unless you have it tested."

Rosemary Gladstar is a staunch defender of comfrey. "The small amounts of pyrrolizidine alkaloids found in comfrey are balanced by this herb's abundance of the cell proliferant allantoin and by calcium salts and mucilage, all of which are nutritious to the cells and serve to counteract the cell-inhibiting actions of the pyrrolizidine alkaloids."

For those who wish to take advantage of the plant's exceptional properties without the risk of liver disease, however remote, PA-free comfrey is available from Herb Pharm (see Resources).

For those who grow comfrey or buy unprocessed comfrey preparations, small quantities are unlikely to cause problems, especially in pets on a natural diet. When feeding larger quantities of untreated comfrey to speed the healing of broken bones or other injuries, add milk thistle seed, an herb whose flavonoids help prevent the liver's absorption of PAs. For external use, comfrey is a category 1 herb; for internal use, it is prudent to place it in category 2.

Echinacea. A powerful immune system stimulant, echinacea has been shown to increase phagocytic (white blood cell and macrophage) activity even after the user stops taking it. Although many herbalists prefer to use echinacea in large doses at the beginning of an active illness, early American and modern German research has shown it to be safe and effective for long-term oral consumption. See page 192.

Is echinacea dangerous? Rumors circulated in Europe after a 1996 German television program claimed that allergic reactions to echinacea caused three deaths. A prominent German scientist investigated these cases and proved that echinacea was not a factor. More than 10 million units of echinacea products are sold annually in Germany, and no allergic reactions have been documented. Between 1993 and 1996, the FDA received eight reports of adverse effects in people who took echinacea, including hepatitis, abdominal distress, and arsenic poisoning. In some cases, the products contained other substances or were adulterated, and the FDA was unable to verify a connection between echinacea and any of the eight reported problems.

Recent speculation that echinacea interferes with conception or poses a risk to unborn children is based on test-tube experiments described on page 106 and is not supported by clinical experience in humans, pets, or other animals. Reports of its long-term use interfering with immune function are based on the incomplete translation of a German clinical study. In the study, an accompanying graph showed a marked increase in phagocytic activity of human granulocytes for the first five days, followed by a gradual drop over the next five days. The translation failed to note that the echinacea was given for only five days, not ten. Echinacea, Europe's most widely prescribed botanical medicine, is an exceptionally safe and effective category 1 herb for pets and people.

Essential oils. Essential oils are so concentrated that tiny amounts of some can harm most pets. Some "safe" oils are especially harmful to pets with epilepsy or allergies. Essential oils should be used with caution during breeding, pregnancy, whelping, and nursing.

Garlic and onion. Like other members of the lily family, garlic, onions, chives, and shallots contain sulfur compounds and volatile oils that have a beneficial effect on the health of pets and people. In 1992, however, the *American Journal of Veterinary Research* reported that onion-induced oxidation of canine red blood cells caused severe reactions in some dogs, including those who consumed small portions of the vegetable. Later reports from other researchers warned that garlic can be hazardous to cats. There is now a great deal of confusion over garlic and onion, which are common ingredients in pet supplements and widely recommended for all animals.

Heinz-body anemia is a potentially life-threatening blood disease caused by the excessive and prolonged ingestion of garlic, onions, turnips, kale, and other plants rich in vitamin K. Scientists speculate that chemical compounds in these plants deplete a naturally occurring glucose enzyme whose special function is to protect the walls of red blood cells. Its depletion causes oxidative damage to red blood cells, leading to the formation of "Heinz bodies," which are rejected from the bloodstream, resulting in dark-colored urine. If this dumping process continues unchecked, the animal can become anemic and eventually die.

The recorded cases of allium poisoning typically involve onion doses exceeding 0.5 percent of the animal's body weight. A dog weighing 60 pounds would have to ingest a 5-ounce onion or several cloves of garlic to begin the Heinz-body process. Red blood cells regenerate quickly in healthy animals, so the overdose would have to be repeated frequently to cause harm. Small amounts of garlic and onion are unlikely to cause problems for dogs and cats on a raw, natural diet, especially if these herbs are fed in courses (see page 123) rather than every day. These are category 1 herbs.

Ginseng. The most famous herb of all, ginseng is often given to athletic dogs, stud dogs, and pets experiencing stress. It is controversial partly because in 1979 the *Journal of the American Medical Association* published an informal poll of 133 psychiatric patients who also claimed to be ginseng users. The patients consumed up to 15 grams of ginseng daily (more than twice the highest recommended dose), inhaled or injected the herb (bizarre applications by any standard), or took it with large amounts of coffee. Most of them experienced symptoms ranging from morning diarrhea to nervousness, insomnia, and elevated blood pressure. All of these are side effects associated with caffeine. It also turned out that some of these patients took "desert ginseng," a laxative, by mistake (it is not a ginseng species). This extremely misleading report continues to be quoted in medical journals as evidence of ginseng's adverse side effects. Ginseng is a category 1 herb.

Hops. In 1995, the National Animal Poison Control Center at the University of Illinois in Urbana recorded eight fatal cases of hops toxicity; the victims were seven Greyhounds and a Labrador Retriever mix whose ingestion of spent hops from home beer-brewing kits resulted in malignant hyperthermia, an uncontrollable fever rising as fast as 2 degrees F every five minutes. Warnings soon appeared in dog magazines, veterinary journals, and herb publications about the dangers of hops to dogs, especially Greyhounds.

There is a world of difference between a bucketful of hops residue from beer making and the small amounts of fresh or dried hops used in herbal teas, powders, and tinctures. Growers, manufacturers, and distributors reported nothing different about their hops production methods when the beer kits were assembled, and the cause of the problem remains a mystery. No cases of hops toxicity have been reported since the original eight cases. Hops is a category 1 herb.

Kava. This South Pacific herb, also known as kava kava, has quickly become one of America's fastest-selling herbs. Kava reduces stress and anxiety, helps focus attention, promotes restful sleep, and relaxes muscles. Large doses, however, have adverse side effects, including a temporary lack of coordination and, over time, an unattractive skin rash. Kava is not recommended for people or pets who are clinically depressed. Although not a mood-elevating herb, kava helps dogs and cats ignore distractions. This is a safe category 2 herb for short-term use in courses (see page 123).

Lobelia. Also known as Indian tobacco, lobelia has a long and colorful history. It is an important ingredient in blends for pets because it causes the immediate relaxation and expansion of contracted parts of the respiratory system, such as the bronchial tubes, esophagus, glottis, and larynx, making it a specific for nearly every respiratory condition. It is also a relaxing nervine, or tonic for the nerves. When blended with other herbs, lobelia acts as a catalyst, increasing their effectiveness.

However, lobelia's nineteenth century promoters enjoyed so much popularity that the medical establishment of the day brought charges against them. Witnesses fabricated testimony blaming lobelia for a host of problems that it didn't cause. The herb's tarnished reputation survives today, with reference books and FDA reports claiming that it is poisonous, toxic, dangerous, and potentially fatal. These accusations, all of which stem from nineteenth-century trials conducted in the United States and England, remain unproven. According to Mark Blumenthal, executive director of the American Botanical Council and publisher of the journal *HerbalGram*, some scientists want to ban lobelia because in large doses it causes vomiting. Blumenthal notes, "It has nowhere near the toxic potential of aspirin or ibuprofen." Lobelia is a safe category 2 herb.

Pennyroyal. Although pennyroyal has been blamed for liver damage, convulsions, comas, and death in pets and people, these adverse effects are associated with its essential oil, which is extremely concentrated, or with the daily administration of pennyroyal tea to infants. Pennyroyal essential oil should be used with caution and is not recommended for use on or around pregnant animals, but fresh pennyroyal and pennyroyal tea can be safely applied to a pet's fur. Its diluted essential oil can be used on herbal flea collars for dogs or applied to a dog's bedding to repel insects. This essential oil should not be used on or around cats. Pennyroyal is a category 2 herb.

Sassafras. A traditional ingredient in spring tonics and a flavorful digestive aid, sassafras contains safrole, a substance that the FDA tested in large quantities on rats in the 1950s. When the rats developed liver cancer, safrole was blamed. Safrole is also found in nutmeg, black pepper, and mace, but these seasonings were never implicated. Because safrole is not soluble in water, someone who drinks sassafras tea ingests very little of it, and no case of liver damage from sassafras tea has ever been reported. The southeastern United States, where most sassafras tea is consumed, has a lower liver cancer rate than other parts of the country. Sassafras is used in some worming blends for dogs and cats, and their recommended doses and schedules are unlikely to cause problems in pets. Sassafras is a category 2 herb.

Tea tree oil. Although widely recommended for use at full strength on pets, tea tree oil is a highly concentrated essential oil. Its topical application has caused temporary paralysis in some animals (see page 186). Like most essential oils, tea tree oil should be diluted before being applied to dogs and *extremely* diluted for use with cats. Tea tree hydrosol (distillate or flower water) is a safer product for cats.

Wormwood. Another plant with vermifuge or worm-repelling properties is wormwood, a member of the artemisia family with a long history of safe use in people and animals. Because wormwood essential oil is a key ingredient in the infamous liqueur absinthe, which was outlawed in Europe and the United States nearly a hundred years ago, some authorities consider wormwood dangerous in any form, warning that it causes convulsions, loss of consciousness, and hallucinations. Fresh or dried wormwood in the amounts recommended for pets has none of these effects. Even wormwood essential oil, which is highly concentrated, is safe for internal use when sold as a flavoring agent from which the psychoactive principles have been removed. Liberty Natural Products sells this type of oil, which is labeled FCC for Food Chemical Codex. Wormwood is a safe category 2 herb.

Yucca. A member of the lily family, yucca has several common names, including soapweed. You can literally wash your clothes—or your dog—with it. The same saponins that give yucca its soapy properties help relieve the inflammation of arthritis, but they also irritate the stomach lining as well as intestinal mucosa. The digestive distress that results from too much yucca can cause bloat, and prolonged exposure to saponins can cause anemia as well as disturbances of the central nervous system. Other foods that contain saponins include soybeans, alfalfa, oats, legumes, potatoes, garlic, and beet pulp.

Yucca is a category 2 herb. It is safe in small doses for most animals but should not be given in large amounts. Avoid administering yucca more than four or five times per week, more than a month or two at a time, or during pregnancy. It is a good idea to avoid other saponin-rich foods when using yucca.

How Toxicity Is Reported

Most warnings about toxic herbs stem not from experience but from theory and the way in which herbs are researched, regulated, and reported. Herbs contain hundreds of chemicals, and it is not unusual for an herb with a long history of safe, effective use to contain one or several chemicals that, when isolated and fed to laboratory animals, cause serious problems.

Toxicologists determine the relative safety of a drug by weighing its benefits against anticipated risks. Aspirin and ibuprofen cause between

10,000 and 20,000 human deaths per year, a statistic that receives little publicity. Most health care professionals regard this finding as unfortunate but acceptable in light of the pain relief these drugs provide. In contrast, herbs used medicinally are so rarely toxic that single cases of adverse side effects make headlines.

Some confusion in the United States stems from the FDA's GRAS, or Generally Recognized as Safe, list, which contains about two hundred herbs commonly used as extracts, flavorings, oils, and seasonings. An additional two hundred herbs in common use do not appear on the list, such as slippery elm bark, burdock root, arrowroot, catnip, coltsfoot, echinacea, flaxseed, goldenseal root, gotu kola, hibiscus flowers, horsetail, uva ursi, stinging nettle, saw palmetto berry, skullcap, senna, tormentilla, blue vervain, and yellow dock root. Such herbs are not unsafe; they are simply unlisted.

The Herb Research Foundation (HRF) gathers scientific data pertaining to herb safety from around the world. If you have questions about the safety of any herb, or if you'd like information about an herb's uses, contact the HRF (see Resources).

Common sense and education are your best guides. Don't use an herb without learning about it first. The safest herbs may be those you grow yourself using organic methods, plants you harvest from areas that are free of pesticides and far from highways and automobile exhaust, and dried herbs purchased from reputable sources, labeled organically grown, or wildcrafted. Unfortunately, most herbs imported into the United States are fumigated on arrival, a consideration for anyone using herbs medicinally. No discussion of herb safety would be complete without a mention of this concern. Check with distributors and importers to learn whether their products may contain fumigation chemical residues.

Interactions

Can one herb interfere with the effects of another? Is it dangerous to mix herbs? What about pharmaceutical drugs? Can herbs interfere with their action or create adverse side effects?

Adverse side effects caused by category 1 and category 2 herbs are extremely rare, either alone or in combination. Allergic reactions can happen in pets just as they do in people, but the herbs most commonly given to animals are not known for producing adverse side effects when combined with other herbs.

If a dog or cat is anxious or frightened, any combination of relaxing nervines may help, but the total dosage should not greatly exceed the recommended dosage of any single ingredient. For example, the animal might be helped by 10 drops of valerian tincture, 10 drops of skullcap, 10 drops of passionflower, or 10 drops of chamomile, or by 10 to 15 drops of a combination of any or all of these tinctures. The same animal could simultaneously be taking a full dose of hawthorn berry extract for heart disease, a full dose of black walnut or other worm-repelling herbs for protection against parasites, and a full dose of joint-limbering herbs for arthritis, none of which is likely to interact in any detrimental way.

The interaction of herbs and pharmaceutical drugs is more complex. Some veterinarians have used herbs and essential oils in orthodox therapies with good results, often reducing or eliminating prescription drugs in the process. For the treatment of serious conditions, medical supervision is always recommended. Herbs that reduce blood sugar levels, for example, may lower a diabetic animal's need for insulin. Castor oil so dramatically increases the skin's absorption that any drug, herb, or chemical applied to the skin at the same time will quickly move into the bloodstream. Herbs that thin the blood, such as garlic and ginkgo, may change an animal's response to anticoagulant drugs. These herbs should be used with caution in animals with blood-clotting disorders. To avoid surgical complications, they should be discontinued before any animal has elective surgery. Both garlic and ginkgo speed post-operative healing in pets that don't have bleeding disorders. In addition, foods and herbs that contain saponins, such as garlic, yucca, soybeans, oats, legumes, beet pulp, and alfalfa, should not be used simultaneously because of potential damage to red blood cells or digestive disturbances.

The *PDR for Herbal Medicines*, an annual *Physicians' Desk Reference* first published in 1998, devotes five pages to possible drug/herb interactions, only a few of which involve herbs or drugs given to dogs or cats:

- Feverfew (*Tanacetum parthenium*), recommended for dogs with arthritis, increases the antithrombotic effects of aspirin and warfarin sodium.
- White willow (*Salix* species), a natural form of aspirin, should be used with caution with non-steroidal anti-inflammatory drugs and salicylates.
- Psyllium husk powder, flaxseed, and laxative herbs can interfere with the absorption of other drugs taken simultaneously.
- Brewer's yeast (*Saccharomyces cerevisiae*), in combination with monoamine oxidase (MAO) inhibitors, may increase blood pressure.
- Medication that increases uric acid levels may decrease the effects of uva ursi (*Arctostaphylos uva-ursi*), an herb used to treat urinary tract infections.
- Long-term use of rhubarb root (*Rheum palmatum*) in combination with cardiac glycosides may increase their effect due to potassium loss.

How to Administer Herbs to Your Pet

If the herb smells suspicious even to you, how are your going to convince Sweet Pea to swallow it?

When it comes to medicinal herbs, some pets are born cooperative. They think everything is a treat. Others walk away, shove the offending substance around with their noses, or scrape the floor as though burying something in the litter box.

One way to make new foods, new supplements, and new herbs palatable to dogs and cats is to expose them continuously to new foods, new supplements, and new herbs. Pets offered an assortment of flavors every day are far more likely to experiment with the new and novel than those who receive the same food at every meal.

Even if a pet dislikes an herb by itself, the herb can be disguised. Tinctures and medicinal-strength teas can be placed in capsules, which can then be hidden in food or given directly. To give your dog or cat a pill, tilt the head back, open the mouth wide, place the capsule over the tongue, then close the mouth and hold it closed. Stroke the throat and gently blow into the animal's nose. In most cases, involuntary muscle reactions send the capsule on its way. Your veterinarian can demonstrate how to administer pills in this manner or with a plastic dispensing tool.

Liquids can be administered orally by making a pouch at the side of the mouth with the lower lip and squirting or dropping the liquid alongside the back lower teeth. It is much easier to administer liquids from the side of the mouth. Another way to give a tincture, tea, or liquid extract is to spray it into the animal's mouth using a small atomizer. The buccal cavity consists of the tongue, teeth, and inside of the cheek, and anything sprayed over its surface will be rapidly absorbed into the bloodstream.

The owner of a lively, distracted young dog in Samantha's agility class asked a health store clerk to suggest an herb that might help her dog relax. She brought a spray bottle of kava extract to the next class and sprayed a small amount into his mouth. Within two to three minutes, the dog was noticeably calmer. Not all herbs sprayed into the mouth will work as dramatically as kava, which is a gentle muscle relaxant that alleviates anxiety and helps improve concentration.

There are several ways to make pilling and squirting less traumatic, such as by offering a treat before and after and by praising, petting, and thanking the pet for her cooperation. It's also a good idea to confine these application methods to preparations that don't have an objectionable taste.

Another option is to avoid the mouth entirely and administer the preparation by ear, as described on page 159. This approach is probably most effective in the administration of nervines, such as valerian, skullcap, oatstraw, passionflower, and chamomile.

Tonic herbs, which should be given daily over long periods, can be added to drinking water and/or food, starting with a few drops of tincture or medicinal-strength tea at every meal and gradually increasing to the desired amount. Over time most pets become accustomed to the taste and accept increasing amounts.

To introduce an herb in food, use food that is itself strongly flavored, like fish, or somewhat sticky, like cream cheese or raw honey. Capsules can also be hidden in pieces of banana, meat, and other foods. Serve the food slightly warm rather than cold because warming releases the food's flavors and aromas. Many dogs and cats enjoy the taste of culinary herbs such as parsley, sage, rosemary, thyme, basil, and garlic, all of which can be added to raw food to make it more appealing.

Most of the herbs recommended in this book are safe to administer to pets in teas, tinctures, capsules, tablets, or simply mixed into food several times daily for several days or even weeks at a time.

Because concentration and quality vary among herbal products, just as the pets and people who take them vary in size, weight, and physical condition, it is impossible to specify a single dosage for best results. If you don't notice improvement after using an herb as directed, your pet may need more. If a tea or tincture smells and tastes unusually strong and fresh, your pet may need less.

As you become familiar with herbs, experiment with small doses of single herbs in tea, tinctures, or capsules before giving therapeutic doses. Try the herbs yourself to discover how they taste and how they act. Record your own and your pet's herbal experiences in a notebook for future reference.

If your pet displays any adverse reaction, such as diarrhea, rapid pulse, dizziness, vomiting, itching, rash, loss of appetite, or any other unusual symptom that seems to result from using the herb, substitute something else. Adverse reactions to the herbs recommended here are unusual,

Suggested Doses for First-Time Use of Any Herb
(Give up to 3 times daily)

Animal's Weight (pounds)	Tincture	Size 00 Capsule	Tea
5 to 10	2 drops	½ cap	1 teaspoon
10 to 20	4 drops	1 cap	2 teaspoons
20 to 30	6 drops	1 cap	1 tablespoon
30 to 50	6 to 10 drops	2 cap	4 teaspoons
50 to 70	10 to 14 drops	2 cap	5 teaspoons
70 to 90	14 to 18 drops	3 cap	2 tablespoons
90 to 110	18 to 22 drops	4 cap	3 tablespoons

but just as people have allergic reactions to different foods and herbs, so can their companion animals. Occasionally an herb may trigger a "healing crisis," in which symptoms appear to grow worse for several hours or a day or two before improving, but this usually does not happen. If an herb seems to trigger symptoms of detoxification, provide the nutritional and herbal support described on pages 94–98 and 203–208.

For most of the herbs recommended in this chapter, the dosages above are conservative and cautious. Depending on the condition (chronic or acute, mild or serious), the nature of the herb, and the product's quality, larger or smaller doses may be appropriate. If an herb is given every day of every week, the body may become accustomed to it and fail to respond as efficiently as it would otherwise. For this reason, many herbalists recommend that herbs be given in courses.

Herbal Courses

When you give a "course," you follow a schedule that allows the body to rest and adjust so that it doesn't become habituated to an herb. One common schedule for herbal courses is five days on and two days off for four weeks, followed by one week off. Another example is the canine arthritis schedule on page 158.

Juliette de Bairacli Levy and other authorities recommend that dogs and cats receive a break from all herbs and nutritional supplements for two days per week. Many follow a Monday-through-Friday "herb day" schedule and take weekends off in combination with a Monday-through-Saturday feeding schedule with Sundays (fast day) off. Keep track of your four-weeks-on, one-week-off schedule on a monthly calendar. These are flexible guidelines that can be adjusted to your convenience. What's important is that your pet not be exposed to the same supplements every day for prolonged periods.

If you are using herbs and other supplements to treat a chronic medical condition such as arthritis or parasites, it is not necessary to suspend all herbs and supplements for an entire week every month. You can substitute different products during that period. Many herbs and supplements have similar effects, and by switching from one to another you continue to treat the condition while preventing overexposure to a single product.

You will soon grow used to thinking in terms of courses, which help prevent potential side effects while ensuring continuing effectiveness. The schedule can be as simple or complicated as you like, using several herbs and supplements or only one or two. What matters is that your pet receives the herbs that improve his health while avoiding the problems that result from too-frequent exposure.

Standardized Products

Few topics have so polarized American herbalists as the controversy surrounding standardized products. Standardized extracts, which are the herbal preparations most similar to pharmaceutical drugs, are guaranteed to contain a specific, isolated amount of an herb's key ingredient. For example, many standardized echinacea extracts contain a minimum of 4 percent echinacosides, which are thought to stimulate immune function. Typical ginkgo extracts contain 24 percent ginkgoflavonglucosides, which are believed to enhance memory, and many St. John's wort extracts are standardized to contain 0.3 percent hypericin, which is believed to be its mood-elevating ingredient.

Despite their official-looking labels, standardized extracts are not necessarily more effective or more "scientific" than crude, whole-plant extracts. Plants are complex, not simple, and medicinal herbs typically contain hundreds or thousands of chemicals. Because they are so complicated, scientists don't know how they work. For example, what scientists regarded as the active ingredient in valerian has changed five times in the last decade.

Most St. John's wort extracts are standardized for hypericin, but new research suggests that an entirely different constituent, hyperforin, may be responsible for the herb's effectiveness as an antidepressant. As a result, some St. John's wort supplements are now standardized for hyperforin instead of hypericin. It is likely that neither hypericin nor hyperforin accounts for the herb's effectiveness in conditions that are not mood-related. St. John's wort can repair nerve damage, such as when the fresh herb or an oil infusion of its blossoms is applied to a nerve-damaging injury and the animal makes a rapid, full recovery, or when the herb repairs damage to the skin caused by burns or other injuries. It was traditionally used as a blood purifier, mild diuretic, uterine tonic, and regulator of menstrual cycles, functions likely to involve still other "active" ingredients.

Standardized extracts were created because of the need for consistent experimental doses in scientific studies. Because their similarity to chemically manufactured drugs has impressed conventional physicians, standardized extracts are often promoted as superior, safer, and more effective than competing products. They may not be. Herb books always mention that in large quantities the consumption of St. John's wort, an invasive weed in the Pacific Northwest, has caused photosensitivity (an allergic reaction to sunlight) in cattle. These books usually warn that St.

John's wort might cause a similar reaction in humans while noting that no such cases have been documented. Recently, however, some clinical herbalists have reported seeing photosensitivity in patients taking standardized St. John's wort extracts, a side effect that disappeared after the patients replaced their standardized products with crude whole-plant tinctures. These reports remain anecdotal but suggest that some standardized products may cause more adverse side effects than their whole-plant counterparts.

James Green, director of the California School of Herbal Studies, does not find this development surprising. "When you pull one ingredient out and throw the rest away, you lose the plant's synergy," he explains. "If you use the whole plant, which has a variety of nutritional components, you experience a gentle process that produces a variety of beneficial effects, and the side effects are minimal, if any. Isolate a single ingredient and you experience all kinds of adverse side effects because the body isn't able to recognize or deal with isolated ingredients."

Green's main objection to standardization is that it places the emphasis on science. "When we embrace standardization because it's scientific," he says, "we accept the notion that science will make things better, and in doing so we disempower ourselves. Herbalism thrives in the home. People should realize that the plants are out there, they're whole and perfect the way they are, and you can go out and identify a plant, harvest it, and make your own medicine for yourself and for your family, your pets, and other animals. You have all the personal power you need to make the finest medicines available, and your result can be a medicine that's superior to anything technology can offer."

How to Judge an Herb's Quality

The best dried herbs are fragrant, flavorful, colorful, and pungent. They don't look like shredded hay or smell like cardboard. These plants are dried at low temperatures with active air circulation and stored away from heat, light, and humidity, the enemies of all dried herbs. The best herbs for medicinal use are grown organically or wildcrafted from pollution-free sources, then handled with care at every step of their drying and storage. By their look, smell, and taste, you can recognize these plants—the peppermint is obviously peppermint, and chamomile is obviously chamomile.

As you evaluate dried herbs, keep these simple rules in mind. The larger the piece, the longer it lasts. Powdered herbs begin to lose their flavor as soon as they are ground. The more a leaf is exposed to heat, light, open air, and humidity, the faster it loses its healing properties and its taste.

In regard to shelf life, most herbs probably should be replaced after a year. The most sensible rule, however, is to look, smell, touch, and taste. Roots and bark hold their fragrance, color, and taste longer than delicate leaves and flowers, yet even blossoms and leaves can retain their herbal identity for much longer periods if properly stored.

Grow Your Own

Most herbs are easy to grow. You will find that nothing compares to your own freshly harvested chamomile, calendula, catnip, lavender, comfrey, echinacea, garlic, valerian, wormwood, yarrow, and other useful herbs. In some cases, the difference between home-grown and commercially prepared herbs is dramatic. For example, so much inferior gotu kola is for sale that your fresh supply will be superior to nearly every gotu kola product on the market. Because most commercially harvested herbs are damaged during drying, storage, and processing, the same applies to many medicinal plants. This tender perennial also makes an attractive houseplant. See the Resources for companies that sell herb plants and seeds.

A Note on Wildcrafting

When Rosemary Gladstar and James Green went into the herb business thirty years ago, United Parcel Service delivered boxes of herbs from mail-order suppliers to fledgling herbalists around the country.

Then wildcrafting captured everyone's attention, and all agreed that the finest, most medicinal herbs come from pristine environments far from busy roads and industrial pollution, for plants that fight for survival in the wild are stronger, purer, and more effective than anything one might grow in a garden or buy in bulk from an importer.

Now UPS is back in the collective herbal conscience, only this time it stands for United Plant Savers. A conservation organization devoted to the protection of rapidly disappearing medicinal plant species, United Plant Savers encourages the cultivation of herbs that are overharvested in the wild, promotes the planting of replacement seeds and seedlings, and recommends the use of common herbs whenever they can be substituted for rare or endangered species. As UPS members know, cultivated herbs can be just as medicinal as anything you gather in the wild. Herbs produce more concentrated essential oils and have a more medicinal effect when grown in conditions appropriate for the species and not overwatered or overfertilized.

If you hike with your dog or enjoy being outdoors, wildcrafting offers many rewards. Many medicinal plants, mostly European imports that have crowded out native species, are abundant and ubiquitous, such as chickweed, mullein, plantain, dandelion, red clover, and most of the plants on any herbicide company's list of lawn weeds. Herbs that grow everywhere can be harvested with enthusiasm; so can endangered herbs that are about to be bulldozed to make way for a townhouse development, road, or shopping center. Walking with a field guide in hand, taking an herb class, or going on weed walks with a local herbalist will open your eyes to the many beneficial plants that surround you.

As you become more familiar with the plants in your area, you may want to contribute to the repopulation of native species by planting seeds or seedlings in the wild. To contact United Plant Savers, see the Resources.

Harvesting, Drying, and Storing Herbs

To harvest herbs at the peak of their medicinal effectiveness, gather them in the morning after the dew has dried but before the sun gets too hot.

Although roots can be dug at any time, many herbalists believe that roots are best harvested in autumn, when their nutrient content is highest. To add fresh, raw roots to your pet's diet, dig them at any time; for long-term storage in tinctures or tea blends, wait until fall. Scrub and rinse roots well, then chop them into small pieces to facilitate drying.

To dry herbs, spread leaves, blossoms, and chopped roots on newspaper, old cotton sheets, drying racks, or paper towels with sufficient space between plant parts to provide air circulation. To dry herbs outdoors, place them in the shade on a dry, breezy day. Indoors, place them where air circulates freely. Although I have a low-temperature dehydrator, my favorite way to dry herbs is to drape leaves and stems over a wooden laundry rack between our basement dehumidifier and an electric fan set on low speed for improved air circulation. Another way to dry herbs is to tie stems together and hang the bundle upside down from a nail. Herbs can be dried in an oven set at the lowest possible temperature, preferably under 100 degrees F. Although you can dry herbs quickly in a microwave oven, this method is not recommended for medicinal herbs.

Herbs are dry when crisp and brittle. When dry, herbs can be packed into glass jars, tins, heavy plastic bags, or other airtight containers for storage. Label each container with the name of the herb, date, and the source. Protect your herbs from heat, light, and humidity by keeping them in sealed containers in a cool, dark place. Properly stored, dried herbs retain their potency for years.

Plant Identification by Latin Name

Like pets and people, medicinal plants have official names and call names, nicknames, or common names. The plant *Zingiber officinale* is more familiar to us as ginger, and *Mentha piperita* is better known as peppermint. Latin names are important to herbalists because they identify plants exactly, preventing the confusion caused by two or more plants that share the same common name or by a single plant that has several names.

The herbs mentioned here are introduced by their common names, which are widely used in the United States. A table showing the Latin names of widely used herbs for pets appears in the Appendix.

Herbal Preparations

Herbs can be given to pets freshly chopped or juiced, dried, or powdered, and in teas, syrups, tablets, capsules, or tinctures, not to mention all their external applications such as compresses, poultices, and washes.

If you are new to herbal medicine, relax. The recipes given here and in herb reference books are flexible and forgiving. If you can't obtain an ingredient, find an appropriate substitute. Quantities are flexible, too. As you gain experience, you will be able to develop your own recipes. When you do, be sure to refer to two or three different herb references for information about each plant so that you have a clear understanding of its benefits, potential side effects, and special requirements.

Even if you aren't interested in making your own herbal products, the following instructions will help you understand how herbs are processed so that you will be able to select and use the best product for your pet.

Simples and Blends

A simple is a single herb. Your cat has been a nervous wreck since the puppy arrived, so you put valerian in his food to help him relax, or the pup bruises her shoulder and you apply arnica. Whole schools of herbal healing have developed around simples, in which a single herb treats a condition until it improves.

Blends are combinations of herbs. You want to unwind after a day in the show ring, so you mix chamomile, skullcap, and peppermint to make a tea. A blend can combine two herbs or dozens of herbs. Chinese medicine uses teas and tinctures that contain ten, twenty, or thirty different herbs, and long ingredient lists are not unusual in European and American herb handbooks.

There are no hard and fast rules in herb blending, but for beginners it makes sense to work with simples until you feel comfortable with individual plants, then begin combining two or three herbs together. If you work with only a few plants at a time, it will be easier to identify any plant that generates an allergic reaction or that is unusually effective. Keep a notebook, for individual reactions vary.

A specific is any herb known for its effectiveness in the treatment of a condition, such as crampbark for muscle spasms or milk thistle seed for liver disease. Specifics can be used alone, in which case they are simples, or combined with other herbs, in which case they serve as the blend's active ingredient.

A catalyst, stimulant, or activator herb is often used in herbal blends to increase circulation and digestion. The world's most widely used stimulant is caffeine, an ingredient in many over-the-counter medications because it helps them act faster. Some stimulant herbs are used alone, but most make up a small portion of an herbal recipe. Lobelia and ginger are examples of catalyst herbs added in small doses to many teas and tinctures. (Despite claims to the contrary, lobelia is safe and effective in small doses for dogs and cats as well as people.) Cayenne pepper is a more powerful catalyst, but its hot taste makes therapeutic doses difficult to take orally. Small amounts of cayenne can be added to food, and some animals seem to relish it. Cayenne can be given in capsules for its own beneficial effects or to enhance the performance of other herbs or supplements taken at the same time. In fact, by giving cayenne simultaneously, it is often possible to reduce the dosage of a therapeutic herb without reducing its effectiveness.

Parts as units of measure. Herbal tea recipes usually are given in parts rather than in tablespoons, cups, or other familiar units of volume. When a recipe calls for 1 part peppermint and 2 parts chamomile, your parts can be anything: a teaspoon, a tablespoon, an ounce (measured by volume, not weight), a cup, or a bucket. The herbal ingredients should be of similar size, usually cut and sifted, crushed by hand, or powdered just before blending.

European recipes measure herbs by weight, which makes measurements more exact, but in the United States, recipes almost always measure quantity by volume. To follow a European herb tea recipe, invest in a kitchen scale that measures metric units (grams and kilograms).

Internal Applications

Fresh herbs. Fresh herbs are plants you grow yourself, harvest yourself, or buy from someone who has done it for you. Freshly cut or freshly dug herbs contain everything the plant has to offer, from enzymes, vitamins, and minerals to essential oils and exotic chemicals. Many herbs can be chopped, shredded, minced, or grated and added to your pet's food with excellent results.

Medicinal herbs, such as mullein for respiratory conditions or echinacea for fighting infection, can be given fresh in food as an adjunct to their use in tinctures, medicinal-strength teas, or capsules. Try to feed a changing menu of fresh, well-pulverized herbs in small amounts as often as possible.

FRESH HERB PUREE

Recommended as a daily tonic for all dogs and cats.

Harvest or buy fresh herbs and rinse or scrub them well. Start with small quantities and add them to your blender or food processor's mixing bowl with other foods. If you have several pets to feed or want to make a large quantity, limit the puree's ingredients to herbs.

Puree the ingredients well and add them in small amounts to your pet's food. If your dog or cat is reluctant to accept new flavors, start with a pinch and increase the amount gradually until you are feeding ½ to 1 teaspoon per 10 pounds of body weight three or four days per week.

Any edible plant can be used for this purpose, such as chickweed, dandelion leaf or root, stinging nettle (young plants in spring), horsetail (very young plants in spring), parsley, cilantro (the leaf of the coriander plant, often labeled Chinese parsley), and/or other edible herbs. Puree them in a food processor or blender.

Bitter herbs such as dandelion aid digestion by stimulating bile production. Cilantro has been shown to bind with and remove toxic metals such as mercury from the body; if given daily for two weeks, cilantro acts as a chelating agent and aids detoxification. Stinging nettle is an excellent all-purpose tonic herb. Freshly cut parsley, sage, rosemary, thyme, chives, savory, basil, oregano, watercress, and other culinary herbs make nutritious and flavorful additions to your pet's food. Freshly dug roots such as dandelion are easy to cut and puree. Burdock root is available in some health food stores and in Japanese markets, where it is known as gobo. The edible blossoms of calendula, lavender, nasturtium, chamomile, and other flowering plants are excellent additions. Any cereal grass (wheat grass, barley grass, rye grass, etc.) can be chopped and added. If desired, add small amounts of fresh or dried gingerroot, cayenne pepper, and/or turmeric as digestive aids.

Refrigerate leftover pureed herbs in an airtight container, and try to use them within a day. Herbal purees made in large quantities can be frozen. Fill an ice cube tray with pureed herbs; when frozen, transfer cubes to a freezer bag or well-sealed container for storage. Thaw cubes as needed.

Herbal juices. Some herbs can be processed in a centrifugal juicer, especially if combined with carrots, apples, or other fresh produce. A few others, such as wheat grass, require juicing equipment that pulverizes and compresses the plant material. Like pureeing, juicing breaks cell walls and improves the assimilation of nutrients. Scrub roots and rinse leaves well before juicing.

CARROT-DANDELION JUICE

Recommended for all dogs and cats for improved digestion, blood cleansing, urinary tract support, and skin and coat conditions.

In a juicer, alternate dandelion leaves and/or roots with carrots in approximately equal proportions. If available, add stinging nettle leaves in a smaller or equal proportion. Add small amounts of this juice to your pet's food or water, starting with a few drops or whatever the animal will accept and increasing to 1 teaspoon per 10 or 20 pounds of body weight per day.

Juice from a centrifugal juicer should be used immediately; juice from a macerating juicer or hydraulic press can be refrigerated for several days. Save the leftover pulp for your pet's dinner, too, as described on page 35.

Many health food stores sell organically grown, hydraulically pressed frozen carrot juice and other vegetable juices. Whenever you pour a glass of juice for yourself, offer some to your pet.

Herbal teas. Although capsules and tinctures are convenient, teas provide an herb's medicinal benefits in a form that is easy to assimilate even when the animal's digestion is impaired. Herbal teas can be added to food or drinking, water, given directly, or applied externally.

To brew loose tea, you need some kind of strainer. Loosely woven bamboo strainers are attractive, but they let so many particles through that they work best with teas made of whole leaves. For smaller pieces, such as cut and sifted herbs, line the bamboo strainer with a piece of cheesecloth or cotton muslin. My favorite strainer is made of fine stainless-steel mesh.

Paper coffee filters can be used, but finely chopped or ground herbs may clog the filter long before the tea is strained. Stainless-steel "tea balls" are widely sold, but if you decide to use one, be sure to fill it less than half full. Dried herbs swell in water, and a full ball will not allow water to circulate for optimum brewing.

If you are making a medicinal tea, most herbalists recommend using loose tea for best results. Tea bags are convenient, but they contain only a teaspoonful of plant material, so you will need quite a few. In addition, they alter the flow of liquid around and through the herbs.

Use only the best quality cookware and teapots. Avoid anything chipped, rusty, or cracked. If you use a wire mesh strainer, be sure it is made of stainless steel. Brew your tea in clean ceramic teapots or glass jars. Obviously, avoid using ceramic ware that might contain lead pigment.

A French press, sold in kitchen supply stores, makes loose tea brewing especially convenient. Most people associate the French press with coffee, but it's a great way to brew tea as well. Press the perforated disc down to strain the brew, and the result is a clear beverage with superior flavor.

Although it's common to make beverage teas by the cup, this is an impractical way to brew medicinal teas. Most herbalists make all their teas, medicinal and beverage, in large quantities, at least a quart at a time and often by the gallon. For pet use, a pint or quart jar is convenient and easily fits in the refrigerator for storage.

Most refrigerated teas last for several days or up to a week. Liquid grapefruit seed extract is a natural preservative; to prolong a tea's life, add 1 or 2 drops per cup before refrigerating. Store tea in glass jars, not plastic containers, and label them with the date and contents.

Always inspect leftover tea before using it. Does it have an "off" odor? Does it look different? Could that be mold growing on the surface? If in doubt, throw it out.

Leftover tea can be frozen for longer storage, although the tea will lose some or much of its potency. Frozen tea is best used within a month. To freeze tea, pour it into ice cube trays. As soon as they are solid, transfer them to a plastic freezer bag. Thaw frozen tea in the refrigerator or at room temperature before adding the tea to food. Frozen cubes can be placed directly in a pet's water bowl.

All of the following recipes call for water, but you can brew tea for your dog or cat using a meat-flavored broth that will make the result far more interesting and palatable. Cover soup bones with cold water, add a few vegetables, and let the broth simmer for an hour or more. Use this broth in place of water in any tea you want your pet to swallow. Alternatively, add a small piece of meat or fish to simmering tea.

Infusions or tisanes. The simplest teas are infusions, also known as tisanes (tee-SAHN). An infusion or tisane is made from fresh or dried herbs and hot water. Chamomile, peppermint, and most other leaves and blossoms lend themselves to this method. A few leaves, such as those of uva ursi, an herb used in the treatment of urinary tract and bladder infections, do not release their medicinal constituents unless simmered the way roots and barks are. Only a few delicate roots are brewed as infusions; one is the relaxing herb valerian, which contains fragile essential oils that would evaporate if the tea was boiled. Infusions extract mucilage, volatile oils, some vitamins, and other nutrients. Water quality is always a concern. For best results, use distilled, filtered, or bottled spring water, not chlorinated tap water. The water should be heated to just below the boiling point.

Proportions of herbs to water for most beverage teas:

- 1 teaspoon dried herb per cup of water
- 1 to 2 tablespoons fresh herb per cup of water
- 4 to 6 teaspoons dried herb per quart
- ¼ to ½ cup fresh herb per quart of water

RECOMMENDED DOSAGES

See the dosage schedule on page 123 for general guidelines regarding the use of herbal teas, capsules, and tinctures. Most of the teas described here are safe and effective in doses of approximately 1 teaspoon per 10 pounds of body weight up to 3 times per day, as needed. Category 1 herbs (tonics, adaptogens, alteratives, and other well-tolerated nontoxic food herbs) can be given in larger doses or more frequently.

These are guidelines, not hard and fast rules. For example, use less of an herb that is dense and heavy, more of an herb that is light and fluffy, less of an herb that is fragrant and in excellent condition, and more of an herb that is old and tired-looking. Everything depends on the quality of the herb and the tea's purpose.

CHAMOMILE INFUSION (Internal and External)

Recommended for dogs and cats for improved digestion and to relieve stress and insomnia. Use externally as an eyewash, wound rinse, and coat treatment.

Pour 1 cup almost-boiling water over 1 to 2 teaspoons dried or 1 to 2 tablespoons fresh chamomile blossoms. Cover and let stand 10 to 15 minutes or until cool to the touch. Strain.

Add this tea to your pet's food or drinking water for improved digestion and to help the animal relax or sleep well. Use as a wash to clean debris from cuts or abrasions, or as a rinse to improve coat condition. Chamomile may temporarily darken white fur, so this rinse is not recommended for very light coats.

To use as a soothing eye wash, strain through coffee-filter paper to remove all plant material, add a pinch of unrefined sea salt (just enough to make the tea taste slightly salty, like human tears), then saturate cotton balls or cotton squares and place them over your pet's closed eyes. Hold in place for several seconds. Repeat as needed.

Decoctions. A decoction is a simmered or boiled tea. Roots and seeds are brewed by this method, though some roots with volatile oils require the more gentle infusion procedure, and some leaves must be simmered instead of steeped. Always check individual descriptions in herb reference books.

To make a decoction, use a stainless-steel, glass, or enameled pan with a tightly fitting cover. Roots, whether fresh or dried, should be cut into small pieces. Use the same basic proportions of tea and water as for infusions.

Unlike leaves and blossoms, roots and seeds can be reused, usually three or four times. As flavor and color decrease with use, you can extend the brewing time or replenish herbs by adding small amounts of new material.

BURDOCK ROOT DECOCTION

Recommended for dogs and cats as an all-purpose tonic to improve kidney function, strengthen and clean the blood, improve skin and coat conditions, and treat arthritis and diabetes.

Combine 1 cup cold water and 1 to 2 teaspoons dried or 1 to 2 tablespoons fresh burdock root. (Fresh burdock is sold in some health food stores and is called gobo in Japanese markets.) Cover and bring to a boil. Reduce heat and simmer for 15 to 20 minutes. Remove from heat and let stand an additional 10 minutes or until cool. Strain.

Add ½ to 1 teaspoon per 10 pounds of body weight to your pet's food daily. Leftovers can be refrigerated for up to one week, but check before using and discard any tea that has an off odor or moldy appearance.

Burdock is one of the best alterative or "blood purifying" herbs, so called because it gradually clears the blood of harmful acids. Because burdock root helps balance blood sugar, it is appropriate for diabetic animals. It is also a tonic for the kidneys and lymph system.

For best results, tonic herbs such as burdock should be used daily for several months or years. Burdock is one of the key ingredients in Essiac tea, described on page 205.

GINSENG TEA

Recommended for older pets, working dogs, stud dogs and cats, animals recovering from illness, and animals under stress.

Combine 1 cup cold water and a small piece of dried ginseng root, about 1 teaspoon in size, in a half-pint or pint jar. Cap tightly. Place the jar on a rack or metal trivet in a large pan, Crock-Pot, or slow cooker filled with enough water to surround the jar without letting it float. Cover the pan and bring the water to a boil. Reduce heat to low and simmer for 1 hour. The rack will prevent the jar from rattling and possibly breaking. This method of tea brewing, which also works well for medicinal infusions, is similar to ceramic ginseng cookers traditionally used in China.

Alternatively, brew ginseng tea as a decoction, as described on page 137–138. The root can be stored in the refrigerator and simmered again; the tea keeps well for several days.

Depending on the type of ginseng root you use, the tea may be dark red or clear. An adaptogen herb, ginseng gradually brings into balance conditions or systems that are out of balance. For example, ginseng has a beneficial effect on the heart and circulation, it nourishes the blood and is used to treat anemia, and because it reduces high blood sugar levels, it is useful in managing diabetes. In general, it is recommended for people and animals with deficiency diseases, lowered resistance, and a lack of hormonal balance. For best results, it should be taken for long periods, such as months or years, although it can be alternated or combined with other adaptogen herbs such as schizandra, ashwagandha, fo-ti, Siberian ginseng (a different species), and astragalus.

Combination infusion/decoctions. Some herbal blends combine ingredients that should be infused (steeped) with those that require decoction (simmering). In general, blossoms, leaves, soft stems, and berries are infused, while most seeds, bark, and roots are decocted. To make a combination tea, start with the parts that require simmering but use the full amount of water required for the combined tea. Bring the tea to a boil, covered, then simmer for 10 to 15 minutes. Remove from heat, add the parts that require infusion, replace the lid and let stand another 10 to 15 minutes. If the tea is a premixed blend containing some herbs that should be infused and some that should be decocted, take half the recommended amount of herbs and brew a decoction; then add the other half and let it steep.

The following tea is unusual for containing two leafy herbs (uva ursi and horsetail) and a berry (juniper) that should be simmered instead of infused. None of these herbs release their medicinal constituents at the low temperature of infusion; they need longer exposure to simmering water. By reading herb handbooks and magazines, you will soon become familiar with which method different herbs require.

UTI TEA

Recommended for cats and dogs with urinary tract infections (UTIs). (See note below regarding pre-existing kidney disease.)

Add ½ teaspoon uva ursi leaves, ½ teaspoon horsetail, and ½ teaspoon juniper berries to 2 cups water in a covered pan. Bring to a boil and simmer over low heat for 10 to 15 minutes. Remove from heat and add ½ teaspoon each cleavers, cornsilk, stinging nettle, and marshmallow leaf. Cover and let stand until cool.

Give frequent small doses of this tea, such as ½ teaspoon (1 dropperful) every 2 to 3 hours throughout the day.

Uva ursi is a specific for kidney and bladder infections. Although often called a diuretic, uva ursi does not increase the output of urine; instead, its antiseptic action cleans the urinary tract. Horsetail disinfects the urinary system and is a specific for infections that cause internal bleeding. Juniper berries are antiseptic and diuretic in action.

Cleavers and cornsilk are soothing kidney tonics and mild diuretics. Stinging nettle is a versatile tonic herb that nourishes the entire system and has such a special affinity for the urinary tract that by itself it has cleared both acute and chronic infections in cats. Cornsilk and marshmallow are soothing, demulcent herbs that help prevent irritation of the urinary tract by the uva ursi and horsetail.

Because uva ursi has a bitter taste, this tea can be mixed with a small amount of vegetable glycerine and given by eyedropper. Extra fluids are important, so encourage your pet to drink more water, and add water, juice, or tea to his food.

To treat acute infections, give 1 drop of echinacea tincture per 5 pounds of body weight in a dropperful of this tea every two or three hours until the infection clears.

For chronic UTIs, give both tea and tincture in five-day courses, but vary the recipe by omitting either the horsetail or juniper berries every other week, as neither is recommended for long-term use. For cats whose UTI is complicated by pre-existing kidney disease, omit the horsetail and juniper berries altogether.

Another herb that helps prevent and treat this widespread problem is the cranberry, which contains chemicals that prevent bacteria from adhering to urinary tract tissue. Although no cat will want to swallow cranberry juice, which is very astringent, cranberry juice extract capsules are popular supplements. Adjust label dosage to your pet's weight. Blueberries were recently shown to have the same effect, making fresh blueberries or blueberry juice an effective alternative.

Medicinal teas. A medicinal tea is a concentrated tea for therapeutic purposes made by increasing the proportion of herbs to water, increasing the brewing time, or both. The UTI tea, given above, is an example of a stronger-than-average tea with therapeutic benefits.

Use up to twice as much plant material as for a beverage tea; the quantity depends on the quality of the herb. If the herbs are potent, you may need less. Let the tea stand until cool or overnight before straining. Store leftover tea in the refrigerator for no more than two or three days. For medicinal purposes, the tea should be strong and fresh.

Another way to brew a medicinal tea is to make an attenuated infusion. I learned this method from the herbalist Billie Potts, who says, "I steep the herb in boiling water, let it stand for three to four hours and then, without removing the plant material, gently reheat the tea at a slow simmer for one hour."

Still another way to improve the effectiveness of a medicinal tea is to brew it in a sealed jar surrounded by water, as described for ginseng tea on page 139. Simmer the tea for at least an hour and let it stand until cool before opening the jar.

To make a medicinal tea more effective, use water to which you have added Willard Water concentrate (see page 87), and add a pinch of unrefined sea salt just before serving.

PARSLEY WATER

Recommended for all dogs and cats as a urinary tonic and to improve the effectiveness of herbs given for parasite prevention.

Add 1 large bunch (the size sold in supermarkets) of fresh Italian or curled parsley to a pan containing 1 quart boiling water. Cover and let stand 3 to 4 hours, then return the covered pan to the stove and simmer over the lowest heat setting for 1 hour. Remove from heat, let cool, and strain.

Add 1 teaspoon tea per 10 pounds of body weight to your pet's dinner daily. For long-term storage, freeze the tea in ice cube trays, then transfer to a sealed plastic bag for storage.

This attenuated infusion of parsley is appropriate for long-term use with dogs and cats. Parsley water is part of a popular anti-parasite program that also uses black walnut hull tincture, ground cloves, and wormwood, as described on page 147.

Tinctures. Tinctures are liquid extracts that concentrate and preserve an herb's medicinal and nutritional properties. These are the preparations you see in the small amber-glass bottles with eyedropper tops that line the shelves of health food stores and herb shops. Because they are simple to use, easy to store, portable, and effective in small quantities, tinctures are very popular.

They are also expensive. Even though doses usually are measured in drops, it doesn't take long for a large-breed dog or a multi-pet household to go through a 1-ounce bottle. How much can you save by making your own? A 1-ounce bottle of black walnut hull tincture made from green black walnut hulls costs between $6 and $10, but for less than $15, I made half a gallon.

Even more important is the product's quality. If you use fresh herbs that you grow or collect yourself, or herbs that have been carefully dried at low temperatures and stored away from heat and light, you can make tinctures in whatever quantity you like. The result will be as good as or even better than any tincture you can buy.

Tinctures usually are made with alcohol, vegetable glycerine, or apple cider vinegar. Alcohol is the most widely used tincture solvent because it extracts more constituents and preserves them longer than anything else. While adult dogs, large puppies, and adult cats may safely take an alcohol tincture, kittens and young puppies should have minimal exposure to alcohol. Health food stores and herb companies offer tinctures from which the alcohol has been removed, or you can buy tinctures called glycerites, which are made with vegetable glycerine. Glycerites are popular among pet owners because their sweet taste makes the tincture more palatable. You can improve the taste of any alcohol or cider vinegar tincture by mixing it with vegetable glycerine or with a small amount of honey, which most dogs enjoy. Tinctures can be diluted in food, water, or juice and given in small doses during the day.

Alcohol extracts fats, resins, waxes, most alkaloids, some volatile oils, and many other plant components. Alcohol tinctures are rapidly assimilated by the body and their effects are quickly felt. Any grain alcohol can be used for tincture making, but it must be at least 25 percent alcohol, which is 50 proof. Most vodka and other grain spirits sold in the United States are 40 percent alcohol, which is 80 proof, and some, such as 151-proof rum and 192-proof Everclear grain alcohol, are higher. High-proof alcohols can be diluted with distilled water if desired, but the percentage of alcohol must remain above 25 percent (50 proof) for effective extraction and long-term storage. The low alcohol content of wine makes it inappropriate for tincture making.

Glycerine is a syrupy, sweet, mucilaginous component of fats and oils from plants and animals. Although inexpensive glycerine is sold in pharmacies, it is a cosmetic item made from cattle bones and far less nutritious than vegetable glycerine. Glycerine dissolves mucilage, vitamins, and minerals but not resinous or oily plant constituents. Glycerites have a long shelf life if stored away from heat and light in well-sealed amber-glass jars. The moisture in freshly harvested herbs will dilute glycerine and thin it slightly, making it easier to pour. If using dried herbs to make a glycerite, dilute the vegetable glycerine with water using 1 or 2 parts distilled water to 1 part glycerine.

Organic apple cider vinegar and other raw, unpasteurized vinegars such as rice or wine vinegar do not break down plant constituents as effectively as alcohol or glycerine, but they extract alkaloids, vitamins, and minerals and are themselves rich in nutrients (see page 77). My teacher, Rosemary Gladstar, recommends vinegar for tincturing tonic herbs, which are slow-acting regulating herbs that should be taken daily to improve the health of body systems, or to revitalize the entire body. Most of the herbal literature warns that vinegar tinctures have a shelf life of only six to eight months, but she has found that vinegar tinctures stored in a cool, dark place last for many years. For best results, use undiluted vinegar containing 5 to 7 percent acetic acid, which is the same strength as vinegar used for pickling. Adding water to a vinegar tincture in any proportion or using fresh herbs that are too moist will cause fermentation and spoilage. Do not use distilled, pasteurized vinegar, which is commonly sold in supermarkets. Look in your health food store for raw, unpasteurized vinegar with a cloudy appearance.

It is easy to make your own tinctures using fresh or dried herbs and either alcohol, glycerine, or cider vinegar. A blend of alcohol and glycerine or alcohol and cider vinegar effectively extracts the plant's medicinal constituents while reducing alcohol levels. By making a double-strength tincture, you can divide the recommended dosage in half, further reducing alcohol exposure. So many commercial tinctures are of questionable quality that your homemade tincture will be superior to many popular brands.

To eliminate alcohol altogether, substitute vegetable glycerine, apple cider vinegar, or a blend of cider vinegar and glycerine. Keep in mind, though, that the result will not be as concentrated as an alcohol tincture, it may not contain some of the plant's key constituents, and its shelf life may be shorter.

The best tinctures have a high herbs-to-solvent ratio, such as 1 part fresh or dried herbs to 1 part alcohol by weight, which is expressed as a 1:1 ratio. If you cover 1 pound of plant material with 1 pound of 80-proof alcohol (about 1 pint), you will make a 1:1 tincture. If you use ½ pound of plant material, your pint of alcohol will make a 1:2 tincture, whereas ¼ pound of plant material in a pint of alcohol makes a 1:4 tincture, and so on. The larger the second number in the ratio, the more dilute the tincture. Tincture manufacturers use hydraulic equipment to extract every available drop of liquid, but you can compensate by letting your tincture age several weeks before straining, by pressing out all the liquid you can, and by using more plant material than solvent.

For the purposes of this book, a regular-strength medicinal tincture is made by filling a glass jar with fresh plant material so that the jar is full but there is room for liquids to circulate. Then, the jar is filled to the top with vodka or other alcohol. If using dried plant material, a regular-strength medicinal tincture is made by filling the jar ¼ to ½ full, covering it with alcohol, and as the dry plant material absorbs the liquid, adding more alcohol so that there is always a 1-inch margin of liquid above the layer of herbs. A double-strength medicinal tincture is made by following either of these methods. After the process is complete, the tincture is strained into a second glass jar containing fresh or dried herbs, and the process is repeated.

The following recipes demonstrate several approaches to tincture making.

BLACK WALNUT HULL TINCTURE

Recommended for all dogs and cats for parasite prevention. The tincture can be applied externally to ringworm and other fungal infections.

If you have access to a black walnut tree in the fall when it begins to drop its nuts, gather fresh green hulls before they begin to turn dark. Wearing rubber gloves (the husks stain everything they touch with a long-lasting dye), pare the hulls with a sharp knife and loosely fill a glass jar with pieces of green hull. Cover the hulls with 80-proof vodka or a blend of vodka and vegetable glycerine or cider vinegar. The liquid will quickly turn dark. Tightly seal the jar and leave it in a warm place for at least a month (longer usually is better in tincture making), shaking the jar every few days.

To make a double-strength tincture, strain the tincture into a second jar filled with freshly cut green hulls and repeat the process. Black walnut hulls will stay green for several weeks if refrigerated.

To protect the medicinal benefits of this tincture, strain it into amber-glass bottles that are filled to the top before capping. This reduces the tincture's exposure to air.

Add this tincture to your pet's food to help prevent internal parasites, including heartworm, and discourage biting insects such as fleas and mosquitoes.

TINCTURE DOSAGES

Well-made tinctures are sufficiently concentrated to be measured by the drop or, if using a rubber-bulb eyedropper, by the dropperful. The dropper in a 1-ounce amber-glass bottle holds approximately 30 drops, which is ½ teaspoon.

In general, begin by giving your pet 2 drops of tincture per 10 pounds of body weight 3 times per day. If using a double-strength tincture, use 1 drop per 10 pounds.

Tincture dosages can and should be adjusted. An animal with a rapid metabolism or serious illness may need more, and larger amounts may be needed if the tincture is not of the highest quality.

Clark's anti-parasite program. Hulda Clark, author of *The Cure for All Cancers*, *The Cure for All Diseases*, and other books, developed an anti-parasite program that is popular among pet owners.

- **Week 1:** Add parsley water (see page 142) to your pet's dinner, using 1 teaspoon per 10 pounds of body weight.
- **Week 2:** Continue the parsley water and add 1 drop of black walnut hull tincture per 10 pounds of body weight, giving the tincture daily to dogs and twice per week for cats.
- **Week 3:** Continue with the parsley water and black walnut hull tincture, and add 1 capsule containing 200 milligrams powdered wormwood per 10 pounds of body weight (several commercial blends contain this amount, while a size 00 capsule of finely powdered wormwood contains approximately 500 mg and should be used at the rate of 1 capsule per 25 pounds).
- **Week 4:** Continue the parsley water, black walnut hull tincture, and wormwood, and add 1 clove capsule (containing 500 milligrams ground cloves) per 10 pounds of body weight.
- Continue with all four herbs for two or more weeks.

As a result of this program's popularity, health food stores offer dozens of preparations combining black walnut hull, cloves, and wormwood in combination liquid extracts, capsules, or kits.

Some pet nutritionists have developed their own versions of Clark's program, adding different herbs, glandular supplements, and other nutrients to support the body as it eliminates parasites. Others have added garlic, which strips mucus from the intestines, making parasites more vulnerable to herbs. Also used are diatomaceous earth, coarsely chopped pumpkin seeds, or seeds from citrus fruit, all of which injure and irritate parasites' soft bodies.

Any herbal parasite program can be given in courses, in which a schedule is followed for a certain length of time, then discontinued or interrupted. For example, the schedule described above could be given to a dog, cat, or other pet for six to eight weeks every three or four months. In between, other vermifuge (worm-repelling) herbs can be substituted, such as chapparal, rue, and pau d'arco. Chinese medicine has its own extensive repertory of vermifuge herbs. Any worm-repelling herb can be given in capsules or added to food. It's a good idea to use different vermifuge herbs on a rotating basis throughout the year.

PERFORMANCE-PLUS TINCTURE

Recommended for dogs in obedience class, agility class, the show ring, tracking meets, and other competitions. This "memory tonic" is also recommended for older pets, including cats, to improve mental function.

Combine equal parts fresh or dried gotu kola leaf, valerian root, and rosemary leaf. Fill a jar approximately half full and cover with vodka and/or cider vinegar or vegetable glycerine. If using fresh herbs, cover them with a 1-inch margin of liquid; if using dried herbs, fill the jar. Leave the tightly sealed jar in a warm place for a month or longer, shaking it every few days, and adding more liquid as necessary.

For daily use, give 2 or 3 drops per 10 pounds of body
weight 2 or 3 times per day.

Approximately 15 to 20 minutes before an event, give
small dogs ½ dropperful (approximately ¼ teaspoon), large
dogs 1 dropperful, and giant breeds 2 dropperfuls.

Alternatively, combine equal parts of commercially produced valerian
and gotu kola tinctures, or use a memory tonic blend that contains these
ingredients. For best results, use a tincture made from fresh rather than
dried herbs, for both gotu kola and valerian are fragile and lose much of
their potency if dried at high temperatures or stored incorrectly. Gotu
kola is easy to grow as a houseplant during the winter and outdoors in
warm weather, and its spicy leaves make an excellent addition to your
pet's dinner.

Gotu kola crosses the blood-brain barrier and stimulates mental
activity. Valerian does not sedate working animals; instead, it improves
their coordination, focus, and concentration. Rosemary is a traditional
ingredient in memory tonics.

Other herbs that help dogs focus and concentrate include ginkgo
and kava, both of which are widely sold in capsules and liquid extracts.
Although ginkgo trees grow throughout the United States, the leaves' medicinal constituents are difficult to extract, and commercial products tend
to be more effective than homemade teas and tinctures. For older animals
and those with impaired circulation, kidney failure, or the early signs of
cerebrovascular deficiency, liquid ginkgo extract is often prescribed at the
rate of 0.25 milliliter to 0.75 milliliter for each 50 pounds of body weight,
two or three times daily. Because ginkgo inhibits platelet aggregation in
the blood, it should not be given to dogs with bleeding disorders, to an
animal that is bleeding from an injury, or for a few days before and after
elective surgery.

Many handlers and trainers are experimenting with different combinations of these key herbs to help their dogs excel. Don't wait until an

important event to experiment; instead, try this blend and others in different settings to find the combination that helps the most. These herbs also may improve a dog's sense of smell.

BONE-REPAIR TINCTURE

Recommended for animals with broken bones, bone injuries, and bone tumors.

Combine equal parts horsetail, comfrey, yarrow, and pine bark to make a tincture, or purchase these tinctures and combine them in equal proportions.

Give 1 drop per 7 to 10 pounds of body weight twice daily.

The October 1998 *Whole Dog Journal* featured the story of Jet, a ten-year-old Belgian Sheepdog living in Australia. Jet's owners refused to have his leg amputated when he was diagnosed with osteosarcoma, an aggressive bone cancer. Instead, they gave him the tincture described above, which was prepared for them by Robert McDowell, an Australian herbalist who specializes in animal care.

Jet's story generated a flurry of phone calls, letters, faxes, and E-mails to and from Australia, not only because bone cancer is notoriously difficult to treat but because the article stated that part of Jet's therapy involved the injection of intravenous horsetail (*Equisetum arvense*). However, this was reported in error; there was no intravenous horsetail, and all of Jet's herbs were administered orally.

Jet's vitality returned, and the shape of his bone mass changed. Nearly a year after his terminal diagnosis, Jet's only complication was a hairline bone fracture that healed with additional comfrey tincture and comfrey poultices, and a photo showed him romping on the beach with friends.

Robert McDowell has shared his bone-repair tincture with canine and feline bone cancer patients around the world (see Resources), and he reports the same promising results in many cases. McDowell makes his own pine bark tincture from freshly cut maritime pine trees, explaining that the popular antioxidant supplement pycnogenol is derived from the same source. If pine bark tincture or fresh pine bark is not available, substitute pycnogenol or other antioxidants.

GINGER GLYCERITE

Recommended for dogs and cats to prevent nausea or motion sickness, improve digestion, treat coughs or sore throats, and (applied externally) to treat minor burns and scalds after the skin has been cooled with cold water.

Loosely fill a pint jar with coarsely chopped fresh ginger-root. Fill the jar to the top with vegetable glycerine, which is available in herb stores and some health food stores. Leave the jar in a warm room for six weeks or longer, shaking it every few days. Glycerine has a sweet taste and viscous consistency that most dogs and many cats find palatable.

To prevent car sickness, give your dog about ½ teaspoon per 20 pounds of body weight 20 minutes before departure, preferably on an empty stomach and preferably without mixing the glycerite with food or water. If your dog is reluctant to swallow the glycerite from a spoon, try mixing it with a small amount of her favorite food. Alternatively, give her powdered ginger in capsules (1 capsule per 20 pounds).

Ginger is safe and effective for cats, though both of mine were suspicious when I tested this tincture on them. However, when I added valerian root, Pepper was eager to taste it. Many cats are strongly attracted to valerian, which is a relaxing nervine and an appropriate herb for any animal who finds travel stressful.

GARLIC-DANDELION VINEGAR TINCTURE

Recommended for dogs and cats as a general tonic and to
help repel parasites.

Loosely fill a pint or quart jar with fresh garlic and fresh
dandelion, coarsely chopped, in approximately equal proportions. Use any part of the dandelion, including roots, leaves,
and blossoms. Fill the jar to the top with unpasteurized apple
cider vinegar from a health food store (the vinegar will have a
cloudy appearance and some sediment) and seal tightly. Leave
the jar in a warm location for a month or longer, shaking it
every few days. Use directly from the jar or strain and bottle.

Add this tincture in small amounts to your pet's food, using up to 1 teaspoon per 20 pounds of body weight per day. This amount of garlic is safe
for adult dogs on a daily basis and for adult cats two or three times per
week. The dandelion is a tonic for the entire body; it helps improve digestion, cleanses the blood, and supports kidney function. If fresh dandelion
is not available, substitute dried dandelion root or leaf, using approximately ¼ the amount of fresh herb.

Unpasteurized apple cider vinegar is widely sold and easy to find.
Less familiar but also appropriate are unpasteurized rice vinegar and wine
vinegar. Do not use distilled, filtered, or pasteurized vinegar for this purpose. Do not feed vinegar or vinegar tinctures to pets who are allergic or
sensitive to vinegar products.

If desired, make a double-strength tincture by straining the com-
pleted tincture into a new jar of freshly chopped dandelion and repeating
the process.

Herbal powders. Because they are easy to administer in food, crushed
dried herbs and herbal powders are popular supplements. For best
results, leave dried herbs whole or in large pieces until needed to preserve
their essential oils and medicinal properties.

An electuary is a powder that is mixed with honey or vegetable glycerine just before serving to improve its taste and make it more convenient for internal use.

Herbs should be stored away from heat and light in well-sealed glass containers for maximum shelf life. When ready to use, grind them in a blender, spice grinder, coffee grinder, or by hand with a mortar and pestle. To reduce exposure to herb dust, which can irritate nasal passages, wear a pollen mask. Store powders in a well-sealed container in a cool, dry place or refrigerate.

SKIN AND COAT POWDER (Internal)

Recommended for all dogs and cats to improve the skin and coat.

Mix equal parts dried horsetail, calendula blossoms, stinging nettle, kelp, and dandelion leaf or root. If available, add dandelion blossoms. Grind small quantities in a spice grinder or blender. Add to wet food, starting with a pinch and eventually reaching ½ teaspoon per 10 pounds of body weight per day (¼ teaspoon for a 5-pound cat, 1 tablespoon for a 60-pound dog, etc.). Maintain this high dosage for a week or two, then reduce to a maintenance dose of ½ teaspoon per 25 pounds every other day.

This powder is similar to the blend of nettle, alfalfa, rosemary, calendula flowers, spirulina, kelp, and dulse developed for pets by Deb Soule at Avena Botanicals, and to Juliette de Bairacli Levy's N.R. Seaweed Mineral Food, which contains seaweed, nettles, rosemary, comfrey, and cleavers. "These herbs are rich in trace minerals," Soule explains, "so they help with a healthy coat of fur and proper pigmentation. The mucous membranes in the body benefit and so do all the organs, bones, and teeth. As a beneficial side effect, these herbs reduce a dog's interest in eating stools."

To help cats accept herbal powders, add a favorite flavor just before serving, such as dried tuna powder or oil from a sardine can. For dogs, add carob powder or something equally appetizing. For any pet with a sweet tooth, mix the powder with a small amount of vegetable glycerine or raw honey.

ANTI-PARASITE POWDER (Internal)

Recommended for all dogs and cats to repel intestinal parasites, heartworm, biting insects, and ticks.

Combine equal parts dried wormwood, cloves (the sweet spice), neem leaves, and rue. Grind and use as described above, or place in capsules and give 1 capsule per 10 pounds of body weight per day for 1 week, then increase to 2 capsules per 10 pounds for 1 week. (One size 00 capsule holds approximately 500 mg; 1 teaspoon is equal to approximately 5 grams or 10 capsules.)

Long used in India as an insect repellent, as a first-aid therapy, and to treat digestive disorders and a variety of health problems, neem has many veterinary applications. In addition to repelling internal parasites, this blend makes the blood bitter and less attractive to fleas, ticks, mosquitoes, and other biting insects.

Neem capsules (see Resources) can be given to dogs and cats at the rate of one 500-milligram capsule per 10 pounds of body weight per day. Powdered neem can be added to food at the same rate. Neem helps combat allergies, arthritis, bad breath, immune system disorders, insomnia, and stress.

DEODORIZING POWDER (Internal)

Recommended for all dogs and cats to improve their natural fragrance and as support during detoxification.

Combine 3 parts powdered wheat grass juice or any other green food (barley grass, chlorella, spirulina, etc.) with 2 parts

dandelion root, 1 part yucca root, and 1 part marshmallow
root. If the herbs are not completely powdered, grind them
in a food mill or coffee grinder. Add to your pet's food,
starting with small amounts and increasing to ½ teaspoon
per 10 pounds of body weight per day in courses lasting
5 days at a time, with 2 days off, for up to 1 month.

Green foods are rich in chlorophyll, which deodorizes by binding with toxins and removing them from the body. Dandelion root improves digestion
and is a tonic for the urinary tract.

Yucca root contains compounds called saponins that inhibit the production of urease, the enzyme that gives ammonia its distinctive odor.
Supplements containing *Yucca schidigera* (Mojave yucca), which is the variety found in most commercial products, have been shown to reduce fecal and
urine odors in dogs and cats, especially those consuming the inferior protein
used in commercial pet foods. Changing to an all-raw diet is itself a deodorizing strategy. Yucca is also known for its beneficial effects on arthritis, psori-
asis, and other skin conditions. However, yucca's high saponin content makes
it inappropriate for long-term use or for high dosages, especially in the concentrated form of tinctures and extracts. Because garlic also contains saponins, suspend the feeding of garlic while using this blend.

Other deodorizing tips for your pet: Brush her teeth (see pages
166–167 and 198), brush a deodorizing powder through her fur (see page
166), use the essential oil coat–brushing treatment on page 182 or the
essential oil–deodorizing treatment on page 208, or try the "sweet breath"
essential oil blend on page 189. See page 166 for dealing with skunk
odors, and see Animal Friends enzyme products in the Resources at the
back of this book.

When dreadful odors overwhelm your pet, the problem may be
solved by a change of diet. Dogs and cats on raw food usually smell much
better than their commercially fed counterparts. In some cases, the cause
may be an illness, so check with a holistic veterinarian if the odor persists.

BLACKBERRY POWDER

Recommended for any pet with diarrhea. Have dried blackberries on hand for use when needed.

Buy or pick ripe blackberries and place them on food dehydrator trays or line cookie sheets with parchment paper, which is sold in the baking section of supermarkets and health food stores. Place the trays or sheets in an oven set to the lowest heat setting. Dry until hard. Store in a glass jar away from heat and light.

When needed, grind the dried blackberries and add the powder to vegetable glycerine, a combination most dogs enjoy, or to small amounts of your pet's favorite food, using ¼ to ½ teaspoon powder per 10 pounds of body weight. Alternatively, fill capsules of a size your pet will swallow. Blackberry powder should help stop diarrhea almost immediately. Repeat several hours later if needed.

Other powders that help reduce diarrhea include powdered psyllium husks, carob, powdered charcoal, and powdered clay, any of which can be added to wet food.

To prevent dehydration, use the electrolyte replacement formula on page 77.

Diarrhea caused by an infectious agent also should be treated with appropriate nutritional support and herbs; see pages 193–196, 198, 204, and 207. Although diarrhea is unusual in healthy pets on a natural diet, dogs and cats changing from commercial pet food to natural food may temporarily experience loose stools. Chronic diarrhea or diarrhea caused by food allergies or digestive disorders should be addressed with the help of a holistic veterinarian.

GENTLE LAXATIVE POWDER

Recommended for dogs and cats. Note that a well-balanced
raw natural diet prevents constipation in healthy dogs and
cats. This powder is recommended for short-term use.

Combine equal parts powdered psyllium husks and apple
pectin. Add ¼ teaspoon powder per 10 pounds of body weight
to enough water, juice, or other liquid to soak it well. As the
powder expands, the liquid will thicken. Add to food once or
twice per day, and give extra fluids.

Sometimes dogs experience constipation as they adjust to a bone-based
raw diet. If raw bones are introduced gradually, this condition is usually
temporary and self-correcting. You also can add grated carrots, grated
coconut, or well-soaked figs in small amounts and ½ teaspoon olive oil,
sesame oil, or sesame tahini per 15 pounds body weight to food.

The herbs cascara sagrada and senna are mild laxatives that can be
used in small amounts. If necessary, add a pinch of either to your pet's
food or water, or use a product such as Swiss Kriss, which contains senna
leaf and other herbs. Adjust label directions to your pet's weight.

SLIPPERY ELM POWDER

Recommended for any pet that is seriously ill or recovering
from an acute illness.

Combine ¼ cup slippery elm powder with 2 tablespoons
acidophilus powder and 1 teaspoon unrefined sea salt. If
available, add the contents of 2 Seacure capsules (see page
90). Add just enough water to make a slippery syrup that
you can feed to your pet by spoon, dropper, or infant
nursing bottle.

To help treat a serious illness or diarrhea, give 1 teaspoon
per 10 pounds of body weight every 2 to 3 hours. For a
vomiting pet, give 1 teaspoon 5 minutes before feeding.

Slippery elm bark is so easy to digest that it has saved the lives of seriously ill cats, kittens, puppies, dogs, and human infants for centuries. Rich in protein, iodine, manganese, trace minerals, and soothing mucilage, this powder reduces mucus discharge, relieves internal inflammation, softens and soothes distressed tissue, heals wounds, protects against infection, stimulates new cell growth, and causes swollen tissues to contract. In addition, slippery elm mixed with water makes an effective wound-healing poultice.

Anitra Frazier credits slippery elm for saving several of her cats. "I would not want to try raising a kitten or nursing a sick cat without it," she wrote in the September 1995 *Tiger Tribe*.

Capsules. Herbal capsules are convenient, tidy, and widely sold. If you need a special blend of herbs, some of the mail-order herb companies listed in the Appendix blend and encapsulate custom orders for a nominal fee. You also can encapsulate your own herbs. Two-part gelatin capsules are sold in health food stores and herb catalogs in sizes ranging from 0 (smallest) to 00 and 000 (largest). For cats and very small dogs, even smaller sizes are available from some distributors. Many herb companies sell mechanical capping devices that hold several capsules in place for faster and easier filling.

If you purchase herbs in capsules, try to buy them from a retailer whose stock rotates quickly or who powders herbs for capsules as needed. Powdered herbs lose their potency when exposed to heat, light, or humidity.

CANINE ARTHRITIS RELIEF CAPSULE PROGRAM

Purchase the following herbs in capsules: alfalfa, boswellia, neem, devil's claw, feverfew, and yucca. For dogs weighing 30 to 70 pounds, try the following per day, Monday through Saturday, in divided doses:

- **Week 1:** 2 each alfalfa, boswellia, and neem.
- **Week 2:** 2 each boswellia, neem, and devil's claw.
- **Week 3:** 2 each neem, devil's claw, and feverfew.
- **Week 4:** 2 each feverfew, yucca, and alfalfa.
- **Week 5:** 2 each yucca, alfalfa, and boswellia.

Repeat the cycle. Alternatively, use 6 capsules of a single herb per day (see the caution regarding yucca on page 117), or devise your own schedule. All of these herbs have an enthusiastic following among owners of arthritic dogs. For smaller dogs, reduce each capsule recommendation by 1, or give a total of 3 capsules per day; for larger dogs, increase the dosage by 1 of each capsule.

Please keep in mind that arthritis is a cooked-food disease, and dogs on a well-balanced raw diet are unlikely to suffer from joint inflammation. The herbs mentioned here work best in combination with a natural diet.

External Applications

Applying herbs by ear. Herbal preparations designed for internal consumption can also be applied by ear. Not many pet owners or veterinarians know about this method, but it works effectively for many medicinal-strength teas and tinctures, especially those that tone and nourish the nerves. Be sure that the liquid is at or close to body temperature. Use an eyedropper to place the liquid in your pet's ear gently (it helps if the animal is lying on his side). Hold the ear closed, massage it, and keep the animal quiet for as long as possible. Even if your pet shakes his head, liquid dropped deep into the ear canal will be absorbed into the body.

This is the method the famous American herbalist John Christopher used to cure epilepsy, as described in my *Encyclopedia of Natural Pet Care*. His B&B tincture (equal parts blue cohosh, black cohosh, blue vervain, skullcap, and lobelia in grain alcohol) applied by ear has treated both people and pets with not only seizures but all types of nerve disorders. One advantage to this method is that it bypasses the digestive process, which can break down some of a plant's medicinal constituents before they reach the bloodstream.

Note: This method is not recommended for tinctures that cause skin irritation or for essential oils.

RELAXING EAR BLEND

Recommended for apprehensive dogs and cats during thunderstorms; when moving to a new home, traveling, boarding away from home or going to the veterinarian; when taking classes or competing; when adjusting to the arrival of new people or animals; when left alone (separation anxiety); or whenever stress is a problem.

Combine equal parts valerian, skullcap, and chamomile tinctures. Using an eyedropper, place 3 drops of this blend into each ear per 10 pounds of body weight. If possible, tilt your pet's head, hold the ear closed, and massage the ear to distribute the tincture.

Repeat the dosage as needed during the day. If desired, dose the animal by mouth as well, using the schedule on page 123. In addition, massage a dropperful of tincture into the skin at the back of the neck.

Other relaxing nervines can be substituted, such as kava, hops, passionflower, or oatstraw, or use Dr. Christopher's B&B tincture (see page 159).

Compresses. A compress is the application of cold herbal tea or a diluted tincture on a saturated towel or thick cloth.

ARNICA COMPRESS

Recommended for any bruise, pulled muscle, or trauma injury in dogs or cats.

Soak a washcloth or paper towel in cold water and apply arnica tincture to it, or add 1 teaspoon arnica tincture to ½ cup cold water and soak the cloth. Hold the wet compress in place with your hand for several minutes or until it feels warm to the touch, then repeat. For best results, treat the injury with arnica every few hours.

The sooner arnica is applied, the more effectively it will reduce or prevent swelling and bruising. If there isn't time to dilute the tincture, such as when an accident happens and all you have is the bottle in your fanny pack, apply it full strength. Use it on yourself, too, when the large stick in your dog's mouth whacks you in the leg or whenever you pull a muscle or bruise yourself.

As described on page 108, arnica tincture is safe for all external applications, including broken skin and bleeding wounds, despite label directions to the contrary. Although large doses can be harmful, arnica tincture can be given internally to stop bleeding and repair the body after serious injury. See pages 108–109. Give dogs 1 drop of arnica tincture per 15 pounds of body weight 2 to 4 times daily, diluted in water; give cats and small dogs 1 drop twice per day. Do not exceed these recommended doses because arnica is a powerful heart stimulant and large doses can cause adverse side effects.

PEPPERMINT COMPRESS

Recommended for dogs with hot spots, fever, heat stress,
or heatstroke.

Brew a strong peppermint tea, which has a cooling effect.
(In an emergency, such as life-threatening heatstroke, pour
cold water over the animal or immerse her in cold water to
begin lowering her elevated temperature; then apply the
herbal compress.)

To cool the tea quickly, pour it over ice cubes. The melting
ice will dilute the tea, so use as much as 2 or 3 tablespoons of
dried peppermint or a large handful of fresh leaves for each
cup of boiling water. Alternatively, add 2 or 3 drops of the
essential oil of peppermint to a bowl of cold water. Vetiver
oil, distilled from the root of the sweet grass plant, is another
natural refrigerant. Either can be used to cool a dog's skin. For
cats, their hydrosols are recommended.

Soak a cloth and wring it just until it stops dripping. The
compress should be wet enough to stay cold for several minutes.

To treat a hot spot, hold the compress in place for several
minutes, then repeat. For the other conditions mentioned above,
apply the compress to the animal's head, neck, legs, feet, or
abdomen and hold it in place. If possible, use several compresses
at once. Circulating blood is close to the skin in the extremities,
making them important cooling points. When the compress
warms to body temperature, soak it again, adding ice as needed to
keep the tea cold. Repeat until the treatment has lasted 15 to 20
minutes. Dry the skin and fur gently.

Hot spots, also known as wet eczema, are unpleasant oozing sores that
often itch and bleed. I used to think that only dogs on commercial diets
got them, but I took a crash course in hot spots when Samantha had an
allergic reaction to the chemicals in a neighbor's swimming pool and
developed one under her chin. A peppermint compress followed by a

fresh comfrey poultice (see page 165) held in place with a thick bandage healed the skin overnight but subsequent itching and scratching broke it open again. Peppermint compresses, aloe vera gel, and lavender essential oil relieved the itching, so I applied these whenever I changed her gauze bandage. I sewed a black cotton wrap with a Velcro closure to protect the wound and alternated comfrey poultices with drying applications of clay powder. The hot spot, which was more than 2 inches wide at its worst, healed within a week and has never returned.

Fomentations. To make a fomentation (hot compress), brew a medicinal strength tea and pour it into a bowl. Wearing rubber gloves to protect your hands from the heat, saturate a washcloth or cotton fabric with the hot tea. Let it cool slightly by exposing the fabric to the air until it is warm but no longer hot enough to scald or burn. Test it on your inner arm to be sure. Fold the fabric to an appropriate shape and size, then apply it to the affected area and hold it in place. Fomentations are sometimes recommended to soothe and help clear impacted anal glands or to bring an abscess or boil to a head to help it drain.

PLANTAIN-ECHINACEA FOMENTATION

Recommended for all pets for infected wounds and abscesses.

To treat an abscess such as a dog or cat might develop after being clawed, scratched, or injured by a splinter or burr, brew a strong tea by pouring 1 cup boiling water over 1 tablespoon dried plantain and 1 tablespoon dried echinacea, or ¼ cup of each if using fresh, chopped herbs. Cover and let steep for 10 to 15 minutes. Strain the tea into a small bowl and follow the instructions above for applying the fomentation, which will draw toxins from the infected wound. Repeat this therapy every few hours until the abscess begins to drain.

Treat a draining abscess with a cold compress or poultice of comfrey, wheat grass, or plantain.

Poultices. A poultice is a wet herbal pack applied directly to an inflamed, irritated, swollen, infected, or injured part of the body. Poultices are made of fresh, mashed herbs or the residue left after brewing tea. They are applied cool rather than hot. Use whatever will hold the poultice in place for as long as possible: bandages, plastic wrap, cheesecloth, muslin, and so forth. A layer of plastic over the poultice helps prevent fabric stains. If the affected area is difficult to treat this way, either because of its location or because of the animal's reaction, put the plant material on folded gauze and hold it in place by hand for as long as the animal will lie still.

Comfrey poultices are an excellent first-aid measure in the treatment of cuts, burns, abrasions, and other injuries. Comfrey contains allantoin, a cell growth stimulant that speeds healing. Practically everyone who works with herbs and animals has a comfrey story, and most involve its direct application.

A widely published warning about comfrey is that it should not be applied to puncture wounds or infected cuts because its rapid healing action may cause the wound to close, trapping the infection beneath it. One herb association recommends that comfrey not be used on broken skin at all. I question this advice because I've used comfrey many times with excellent results, such as when my husband's hand was badly swollen from a spider bite or when a cat scratch on my hand became infected. The husband of an acquaintance cut his hand open with a power saw and was far from a hospital, so he chewed fresh comfrey, applied it to his hand, and tied it in place with a bandanna. The next morning his skin had healed without infection, pain, or swelling; his only inconvenience was having to pull out the small bits of comfrey embedded in the scar. After a friend was pulled head-first down a flight of concrete steps by a visiting dog, she used comfrey on her badly abraded face and recovered quickly. When Samantha sliced her paw pad on broken glass, I wrapped her foot in a comfrey poultice and the wound closed overnight. It may be a good idea to use herbs other than comfrey on deep puncture wounds, but comfrey is an important first-aid treatment for most injuries.

COMFREY POULTICE

Recommended for all animals with cuts, abrasions, bites, stings, and infected wounds (see note on page 164).

If you have a comfrey plant, cut off a leaf, rinse it in cold water to clean it, then chop the wet leaf and grind it in a blender or food processor, or mince it with a knife.

If fresh comfrey is not available, soak dried comfrey in water for several minutes until it rehydrates. Blend the dried comfrey leaf with water in a blender or food processor if desired, or mix them together in a cup. Alternatively, brew comfrey tea and use the residue as your poultice.

Place the soft, wet comfrey mass on a piece of gauze, fabric, paper towel, or bandage, then apply it to the bite, wound, cut, burn, or abrasion. Depending on the injury and your pet's condition, hold it in place with a bandage or your hand for as long as possible. Change or replace the poultice after a few hours or overnight.

Any plant can be used as a poultice, but green plants seem to have a special affinity for infections and toxins. Plantain (the common lawn weed, not the banana) and wheat grass are good examples. A friend treated an infected dog bite on his leg by putting fresh wheat grass through a juicer, recombining the juice and pulp, and holding it in place with bandages. He did this only once and the bite healed quickly without leaving a scar. Horsetail, cayenne pepper, and yarrow are known for their styptic properties; they stop bleeding on contact and are important first-aid poultice ingredients.

Powders. Prepare herbal powders as described on pages 152–155 or remove powdered herbs from capsules as needed. Powdered herbs can be mixed with small amounts of water, tea, or oil to form a paste that can be applied to cuts or wounds.

DEODORANT POWDER (External)

Recommended for dogs with unpleasant-smelling
skin and fur.

Mix together 1 part whole cloves, 1 part broken
cinnamon sticks or powdered cinnamon, 2 parts myrrh
gum (a tree resin), 2 parts dried thyme, 6 parts coriander
seeds, and 8 parts dried lavender blossoms. Grind these
ingredients as needed and sprinkle the powder on your
pet's bedding or rub it into your dog's fur and brush it
out. Because of the powder's dark color, this treatment
is not recommended for white-coated dogs.

This deodorant powder does not address the nutritional cause of unpleasant odors, and it will not neutralize skunk odors.

To treat skunk odors and other formidable olfactory challenges, such as a dog that has rolled in something nauseating to the senses, combine 1 quart of 3 percent hydrogen peroxide with ¼ cup baking soda and 1 teaspoon liquid soap. Apply the mixture to the animal's skin and fur and rinse thoroughly. This simple formula, developed by Illinois chemist Paul Krebaum, immediately neutralizes thiols, the chemicals that give skunk spray, decaying fecal matter, and decomposing flesh their distinctive odors. Because the mixture is too volatile to store, it must be prepared just before using.

TOOTH AND GUM POWDERS

Recommended for dogs and cats. Although raw meaty bones
are effective tooth and gum cleaners, pets that have been on
commercial food often need additional help.

Part 1 ingredients: powdered bee propolis, powdered grapefruit seed extract from capsules, powdered rhubarb juice (see Pines International in the Resources), powdered neem, or powdered mastic. These ingredients disinfect, deodorize, and fight infection, and all are specifics for gum disease.

Part 2 ingredients: powdered clay (pink, green, or white) or powdered charcoal. These carrier ingredients have a mild scrubbing action and are widely used in tooth powders.

Combine one or two of the part 1 ingredients with one or both of the part 2 ingredients in approximately equal proportions. If desired, add a small amount of baking soda or unrefined sea salt, both traditional tooth scrubbers. Moisten a dog or cat toothbrush or a piece of gauze wrapped around your finger with aloe vera juice or gel, dip it into this powder, and massage it over your pet's teeth and gums.

See also the highly effective tooth and gum treatment on page 198, which combines pitch and lavender oil.

Washes and rinses. These preparations are just what they sound like. Any beverage or medicinal-strength tea can be used to flush a cut or rinse debris from a wound or abrasion. Teas can be used as a final rinse after shampooing or even in place of soap.

When my husband's first red tabby kitten began to scratch the furniture instead of his scratching post, I filled a small squirt gun with water and spritzed his back to discourage this behavior. To my surprise, Pumpkin turned, delighted, and begged for a shower. Every week from then on, I brewed a strong chamomile tea (recommended for blondes and redheads), filled a hydraulic sprayer, spread towels on my lap, and soaked him to the skin while he purred and kneaded. A thorough towel drying and an hour in the sun returned his sweet-smelling coat to its fluffy, dander-free glory.

NETTLE COAT RINSE

Recommended for dark-coated dogs and cats to improve coat condition.

Brew an infusion by pouring 2 cups boiling water over 2 to 3 tablespoons dried nettle or up to ½ cup fresh nettle. Cover and let stand until cool. Strain. After bathing (or in place of bathing), gently work the tea into your pet's coat, wetting the skin. Let the coat air-dry.

Vinegar tinctures for external use. Apple cider vinegar is an important food supplement, but it can be used externally as well. Applied to cuts, wounds, hot spots, dull fur, skin infections, calluses, and itchy areas, it soothes the skin, improves the coat, and repels fleas and ticks.

CIDER VINEGAR SKIN AND COAT TONIC (External)

Recommended for all dogs and cats, except those with white or very light fur, to improve coat condition, rinse wounds, heal sores, repel insects, and soothe irritated skin.

Combine any of the following, fresh and/or dried: rosemary leaves, calendula blossoms, rose petals, juniper berries, lavender stalks or flowers, lemon peel, sage, comfrey, plantain, and chamomile. If using fresh comfrey leaves, let them wilt before using to reduce their water content.

Arrange the plant materials loosely in a glass jar (fill the jar only ⅓ full if you are using dried herbs) and cover to the top with unpasteurized apple cider vinegar. Seal tightly and leave the jar in a warm place, in or out of the sun, for 2 weeks or longer.

Strain the liquid through cheesecloth into a large measuring cup. Transfer to storage bottles. Store in a cool, dark place. Shake well before using.

To use as an insect repellent, pour a small amount onto a damp washcloth and wipe your pet's coat. To treat any itch, rash, or irritated skin condition, apply directly. Use this vinegar to disinfect cuts, abrasions, and other wounds. Dilute it with an equal quantity of water for use as a final rinse after bathing your pet and let the coat air-dry.

Oil infusions. To make an oil infusion for treating wounds or ear infections or in preparation for salve making, you can use the stove, the oven, the sun, or an electric cooker. Although any carrier oil can be used, olive oil is the standard for medicinal infusions. Because pesticide residues and other chemicals are easily absorbed through the skin, it's worth investing in organically grown, cold-pressed (rather than chemically extracted) carrier oils.

Cover the plant material with oil and heat it gently in the top of a double boiler above simmering water, in a closed glass jar set on a rack in a pan of simmering water, in a covered baking dish in an oven set to low heat (200 to 250 degrees F), or in an electric cooker such as a Crock-Pot, until the oil assumes the fragrance, taste, and color of the herbs. If using dry herbs, additional oil may be needed as the plant matter absorbs it. Use enough oil to cover the herbs well but not so much that your result is weak and ineffective. Start with 2 or 3 cups oil to 1 cup dried herbs and adjust the proportions as desired. Fresh herbs, which should be allowed to wilt before using, will absorb less liquid, so simply cover them with oil.

To make a solar infusion, let fresh plant material wilt to reduce its water content, then loosely pack a clean glass jar with fresh herbs (or half-fill a jar with loosely packed dried herbs), then fill it to the top with oil. Wipe the rim of the jar clean. Put the lid on tight and leave the jar in the hot sun for several weeks or even months.

When it is ready to use, strain the oil through cheesecloth and add several drops of tea tree oil or grapefruit seed extract as a disinfecting preservative. Pour into a clean glass jar, label with ingredients and date of preparation, and store away from heat and light. Stored correctly, oils can last for years, though most herbalists prefer to make them annually for maximum freshness. Note that these oils are for external use only. Discard any oil that becomes rancid.

MULLEIN-GARLIC EAR OIL (External)

Recommended for dogs and cats with ear infections or inflammation, or to prevent ear infections in floppy-eared dogs or dogs that swim.

If mullein grows in your area, collect its small yellow blossoms after the morning dew has dried and let them wilt in the shade for an hour or two. Otherwise, use dried blossoms. For every loosely packed cup of fresh blossoms or ½ cup of dried blossoms, add 3 to 5 coarsely chopped garlic cloves. Cover the blossoms and garlic with olive oil, wipe the jar rim, and tightly seal with a clean lid. To make a solar infusion, leave the jar in the hot summer sun for a week or longer. Otherwise, place the jar on a rack in a pan of boiling water and simmer over low heat for at least an hour.

Note: This oil is for external use only. Because garlic can harbor botulism bacteria, the FDA requires manufacturers of garlic and olive oil products to add acidifying ingredients such as vinegar or lemon juice. Oil blends containing garlic are safe for external use, and the addition of tea tree oil or grapefruit seed extract as a preservative destroys any botulism that might be present.

For a more effective ear oil, strain the infusion into a second jar loosely filled with mullein blossoms and repeat the process. The most highly regarded ear oil is a triple oleate, made by completing this process three times.

Strain the finished oil into dropper bottles for easy dispensing. If desired, add 5 to 10 drops of tea tree oil and/or liquid grapefruit seed extract to each ounce of oil. To treat or prevent an ear infection, warm the dropper bottle in hot water until it reaches body temperature. Place several drops in your pet's ears (larger ears require more) and massage the ears gently, holding the ear flaps closed; then let your pet shake her head.

If the discharge in your pet's ears looks gritty, like dried coffee grounds, and if the ear looks inflamed and your cat scratches her ears when you rub them or your dog shakes his head and scratches his ears frequently, ear mites are the likely culprit. Vegetable oil–based ear oils are not always effective in the treatment of ear mites, possibly because the oil contains nutrients that feed these tiny parasites. Herbalists take a dim view of mineral oil, which is a petroleum product, because it is poorly absorbed by the skin. In the case of ear mites, though, this trait is an advantage. Mineral oil effectively smothers ear mites and prevents the growth of new generations if applied once or twice per week for two or three weeks. Wipe away any oil that spills on your pet's fur and, if necessary, clean the area with a mild soap or pet shampoo.

ALL-PURPOSE SKIN OIL

Recommended for dogs with skin conditions, burns, cuts, paw pad irritations caused by de-icing salt, abrasions, and other wounds.

If possible, use fresh calendula and St. John's wort blossoms and comfrey leaves that have been left to wilt for several hours; otherwise, use dried herbs. Cover herbs with olive oil, filling the jar to the top. Clean the rim, tightly seal, and leave the jar in the hot summer sun for several weeks before straining. The unusually potent healing properties of this oil, which is colored a deep red by the St. John's wort, may be due to its prolonged photosynthesis or to some magical effect of continual sunlight and moonlight.

Any combination of these three herbs will work well, so if you don't have equal quantities, use whatever is available. The more comfrey you use, the darker green the oil will be; the more calendula, the more gold or yellow; and the more St. John's wort blossoms you use, the deeper red. If fresh herbs are not available, use approximately 1 part dried herbs to 3 parts olive oil and add oil as necessary.

If time and sunlight are in short supply, place the tightly sealed jar on a rack in a pan of boiling water and simmer for at least an hour.

Herbal salves. To turn an herbal oil into an herbal salve, just add beeswax. One of the best all-purpose salves you can make begins with the infusion described above. In addition, every medicine cabinet should have a plain deep green comfrey salve for wound healing.

BASIC SALVE RECIPE

Recommended for all pets with cuts, burns, and wounds.

Combine 1 cup infused all-purpose oil (see preceding page) with ¼ teaspoon tea tree oil, ½ teaspoon grapefruit seed extract, several drops essential oil (lavender or other) and 1 ounce beeswax in a double boiler or over very low heat until the beeswax has melted. Test the salve by placing a spoonful in the refrigerator for a minute. The salve should be soft but not runny. If it's too soft, add more beeswax; if too hard, add more oil. Pour into clean baby food jars or other containers. Herbal supply catalogs sell small tins for storing salve.

This antiseptic, analgesic, soothing salve speeds the healing of cuts, burns, and other wounds. Cats tend to dislike the fragrance of tea tree and lavender, and many dogs are attracted to the olive oil in salve and lick it off as fast as you put it on. None of these ingredients is harmful if swallowed in the amounts given here, although it would be prudent to omit the tea tree oil in a salve that's likely to be swallowed by infant puppies or very small pets.

Even if the salve stays in place for only a short time, it will speed the healing of most skin conditions.

Herbal creams. Oil and water don't mix—unless you whip them together at high speed with both solutions at room temperature. Using the same procedure that makes mayonnaise from an egg and olive oil, you can make a soothing emollient cream that can be applied to cuts, burns, abrasions, and calluses.

Follow the instructions below with care. If your blend separates instead of holding together like a fine face cream, it is still therapeutic; simply shake well before using.

EMOLLIENT CREAM

Recommended for dogs to treat burns, abrasions, elbow calluses, scars, and scratches.

Brew a strong (medicinal-strength) tea using fresh or dried comfrey, calendula, chamomile, St. John's wort, and/or plantain leaves. Let cool.

Measure ⅔ cup tea and add ⅓ cup aloe vera juice or gel and 15 drops grapefruit seed extract. You will have 1 cup liquid altogether. Set aside.

In a separate 2-cup glass measuring cup, combine 2 tablespoons neem seed oil, ⅛ cup castor oil, and enough jojoba, apricot kernel, almond, or olive oil—or, even better, an infused herbal oil such as comfrey, calendula, or St. John's wort in jojoba or olive oil—to measure ¾ cup oil altogether.

To the oil mixture, add ⅓ cup coconut oil or cocoa butter, 1 teaspoon lanolin, and ½ ounce chopped or grated beeswax. Set the measuring cup in a pan filled with just enough simmering water to surround the cup. The cup is a makeshift double boiler that gently warms the oils and melts the beeswax. As soon as the beeswax has melted, set aside to cool. When the oil mixture is close to room temperature, add 20 drops of lavender, sandalwood, or tea tree essential oil, 10 drops of cinnamon or thyme oil, or any essential oil or combination of oils you would like to use.

(Continued top of next page)

(Emollient Cream–continued from page 173)

When the tea/aloe vera mixture and the oil mixture are both at room temperature, place the tea/aloe vera mixture in a blender or food processor. If your food processor has a whip attachment for beating egg whites, use it; otherwise, use the pureeing blade. If using a standard blender, set it on high speed; if using a Vita Mix blender, use low speed. In a slow, thin drizzle, gradually pour the oil mixture into the vortex formed at the center of the swirling tea.

If all goes well, the oil and water will combine in a white cream that holds its shape and doesn't separate. As this begins to happen, add the oil at a faster rate. When most of the oil has been added, watch the cream carefully and listen to the blender. As soon as the blender coughs and chokes and the cream looks as thick as buttercream frosting, turn the blender off. Do not overbeat! The cream will thicken slightly as it stands.

Pour the cream into clean, small jars, such as baby food jars. Label and store in a cool place.

This versatile formula, based on a recipe developed by my mentor, Rosemary Gladstar, does double duty as a superior-quality face cream for people. As she says, "This recipe is a basic formula and is ready for all your enthusiastic ideas: vitamins A, D, and E, elastin, collagen, avocado oil, various combinations of essential oils, herbs, and so on. One caution: It is best to experiment in small batches."

Essential Oils and Aromatherapy

Most people associate aromatherapy with perfume, but the use of essential oils is also a branch of medicine. The volatile oils that give plants their fragrance can be extracted, usually by steam distillation, to concentrate and preserve their substance. The resulting essential oils have profound physical, mental, and emotional influences.

Product quality is an important consideration in therapeutic aromatherapy. Because essential oils are expensive and difficult to produce, many are of inferior quality, adulterated with synthetic ingredients, or mislabeled. Poor-quality essential oils can cause adverse side effects, or they may simply be ineffective.

Thanks to the growing popularity of aromatherapy, it is possible to find hundreds of pure, superior-quality essential oils along with instructions for their use (see Resources).

Those instructions, however, can be contradictory. While writing *The Encyclopedia of Natural Pet Care*, I followed the veterinary guidelines of Nelly Grosjean, a respected French aromatherapist. I have since learned that more dilute concentrations and smaller doses produce good results with less risk of adverse side effects. The doses recommended by Grosjean are most appropriate for healthy animals on a natural diet and for older pets that have been exposed to essential oils all their lives. For other animals, those doses can be reduced by half or more. If you have *The Encyclopedia of Natural Pet Care*, consider using one-fourth or one-half the doses recommended in its aromatherapy chapter. Because therapeutic-quality oils are expensive, this approach is economical as well as safe and effective.

A growing number of aromatherapists who work with pets recommend the use of hydrosols. Also known as flower waters or steam distillates, hydrosols are a byproduct of essential oil production. Lavender water, orange blossom water, and rose water are familiar examples. Although extremely dilute, they retain the fragrance and other water-soluble components of the leaves, roots, or blossoms that produced them, and they contain significant healing properties. Although they do not require refrigeration, hydrosols should be stored away from heat and light. To avoid contamination, open the bottle infrequently. Hydrosols are often sold in 200-milliliter bottles (slightly less than 7 fluid ounces) or by the cup (8 ounces) or pint (16 ounces). They can be poured into dropper bottles or spray bottles for daily use. Do not use a hydrosol that has an "off" odor or contains particulate matter.

"Dogs can tolerate some full-strength essential oils and most diluted essential oils," says aromatherapist Suzanne Catty, "but cats are entirely different. With their thin skin and sensitive metabolism, cats absorb essential oils so rapidly that they can be dangerous. For example, peppermint and spearmint oils, which are well tolerated in low doses by dogs, can be neurologically toxic to cats and cause spasms in the bronchioles."

Aromatherapist Kristin Leigh Bell agrees. "I know someone who diluted one drop of a peppermint oil blend and applied it to her cat's abdomen at the recommendation of an essential oil distributor," she says. "The cat soon displayed symptoms of poisoning and spent several days in the hospital. I am very concerned about multi-level marketing companies that train distributors to use full-strength essential oils on people, horses, dogs, and cats as though we are all the same. We're not."

Substituting hydrosols for essential oils is the only safe way to use aromatherapy for cats, kittens, very small dogs, pregnant dogs, young puppies, and seizure-prone dogs.

Because they are far less expensive than essential oils, hydrosols make aromatherapy more affordable, and their dilution makes even "dangerous" oils safe for all pets. While most retailers avoid hydrosols because of their bulk and cool-storage requirements, some aromatherapy companies sell up to fifty different flower waters (see Resources). Hydrosols are the fastest-growing segment of the aromatherapy market, and this is very good news for pet owners.

Administering Essential Oils

Essential oils are so concentrated that they are measured by the drop. Some essential oil bottles dispense one drop at a time, or you can use an eyedropper. When following a recipe that calls for a teaspoon or fraction of a teaspoon, don't rely on your tableware because teaspoons vary in size, and don't try to estimate fractions. Use metal measuring spoons sold for kitchen use, and test them with drops of water. One teaspoon equals 60 drops.

Essential oils can be administered in several ways. They can be released into the air with an apparatus called a diffuser (available from aromatherapy companies), sprayed into the air from a spray bottle, dropped onto a ceramic or paper ring (another aromatherapy supply) that is warmed by a lightbulb, or simply dropped onto a cold lightbulb that, when turned on, releases the fragrance. Deodorant, antiseptic, and respiration-enhancing oils, such as bergamot, cedarwood, clary sage, cypress, eucalyptus, juniper, lavender, neroli, patchouli, and sandalwood are commonly used in this manner, although heating an essential oil may destroy some of its properties. When sprayed or diffused at cool temperatures, essential oils and hydrosols such as bergamot, eucalyptus, juniper, oregano, and tea tree can help disinfect an entire room, eliminating bacteria, viruses, fungi, and molds as well as unpleasant odors. Diffused oils and hydrosols help animals cope with stress (examples include basil, chamomile, lavender, and melissa), breathe more easily (black pepper, eucalyptus, frankincense, lavender, myrrh, and peppermint), focus their attention (basil, cardamom, peppermint, and rosemary), relax and sleep (chamomile, lavender, neroli, rose, and sandalwood), or overcome depression (basil, bergamot, chamomile, lavender, melissa, neroli, rose, sandalwood, and ylang ylang).

Dilution is the key to making most essential oils safe for use with pets. Cinnamon is one of several essential oils that can literally burn the skin. Undiluted tea tree oil has caused temporary paralysis in animals. Pennyroyal oil can cause potentially fatal liver damage in dogs and cats. Peppermint and spearmint oils, even when diluted, can be toxic to cats. Adverse reactions are sometimes blamed on an oil's quality, but small animals have such sensitive systems that even the highest-quality oils can cause problems.

Only a few essential oils are so well tolerated that they can be applied neat (full strength) on dogs. One is lavender, which has so many uses that it is a first-aid kit in a bottle. It disinfects wounds, heals burns, deodorizes, improves digestion, relieves pain, calms the animal, and neutralizes the venom in spider and insect bites and stings. When Samantha was stung on her nose, a single drop of lavender oil reduced the swelling in minutes. Cuts, burns, and bites can be treated with a few drops of full-strength lavender oil. Lavender oil can be applied to a dog's spine (see page 208) to support detoxification and applied to the feet to calm nerves and improve digestion. It is important to use only therapeutic-grade lavender oil for this purpose.

Another exceptionally safe essential oil is sandalwood. One of the world's most popular fragrances, sandalwood lifts depression and has a relaxing influence in addition to being a gentle but effective antifungal, antibacterial, antiviral disinfectant. Sandalwood essential oil can be applied to skin infections, ringworm, and other skin problems. It can be added to shampoo or used in rinse water to leave a pleasant scent in an animal's coat. The worldwide shortage of slow-growing sandalwood trees will make this essential oil increasingly rare and expensive, so consider putting some aside for yourself and your companion animals. Be sure it comes from a reliable source, because its high cost will make counterfeit and poor-quality sandalwood oil increasingly common. Sandalwood hydrosol makes an excellent substitute.

Chamomile essential oils, derived from the German annual *Matricaria chamomilla* and the Roman perennial *Anthemis nobilis*, have anti-inflammatory, pain-relieving properties and are topical disinfectants that prevent infection, speed the healing of wounds, and improve digestion. German chamomile oil is deep blue in color, but the color fades as the oil evaporates.

Diluting essential oils in carrier oils. Carrier oils, also called fixed oils, are derived from seeds, nuts, or oily fruits. Carrier oil blends are less appropriate for use on cats than dogs because of their smaller size, raspy tongues, and industrious grooming habits. Ear oils (see page 170) can safely be dropped into a cat's ears, but body massage oils are not recommended.

Several effective carrier oils can be purchased from health food stores and aromatherapy supply companies, including almond (sometimes labeled sweet almond), apricot kernel, peach kernel, olive, grapeseed (not to be confused with grapefruit seed), corn, hazelnut, walnut, safflower, soya, and sunflower. For best results, use organically grown, cold-pressed carrier oils, for chemical residues accompanying any oil will be absorbed by the skin. Some carrier oils are best used in small amounts, accounting for no more than 10 to 20 percent of the carrier oil blend; these include avocado, borage seed, evening primrose seed, neem seed, sesame seed, and wheat germ oils. Carrot seed oil, which is itself an essential oil, belongs to this category. Mineral oil, the main ingredient in baby oil, is not recommended.

Castor oil, which has its own therapeutic properties, deserves special consideration because it is so effectively absorbed that it increases the potency of other ingredients. In fact, castor oil is sometimes used to deliver prescription drugs through the skin. When taken internally, such as when it is licked off, castor oil is a laxative, a consideration when treating areas a dog can easily reach. Castor oil's antifungal properties help the treatment of ringworm and similar infections with or without the addition of fungus-fighting essential oils. In addition, castor oil has a special affinity for the eyes and is an effective treatment for styes, conjunctivitis, and other conditions. For medicinal applications, use pharmaceutical-grade castor oil, sometimes labeled triglyceride castor oil. Although water-soluble sulfated castor oil, traditionally known as Turkey red oil, is not recommended for full-strength medicinal use, it is the key ingredient of Willard Water extract (see page 87), which has long been proven to have no adverse effect on pets or people. Some of the world's finest bath oils are made with only two ingredients, sulfated castor oil and an essential oil such as lavender or rosemary. I know of no reason to avoid the use of sulfated castor oil in water-based aromatherapy products for pets.

Jojoba is another carrier with a special affinity for the skin. More properly labeled a liquid ester, jojoba absorbs quickly and carries blended essential oils effectively into the body. Pure jojoba is nonallergenic and does not stain or turn rancid. Jojoba can be used as a base liquid for herbal oil infusions, as a carrier for essential oils, and as a base for creams and massage oils. For best results, use a chemical-free jojoba such as from the Boston Jojoba Company (see Resources).

Amaranth oil, extracted from amaranth grain, can be used alone or added to oil blends to prevent itching and treat burns, rashes, hot spots, flaking skin, and wounds. Its repairs skin and helps prevent scarring.

There is no single formula for diluting essential oils in carrier oils. In *The Complete Book of Essential Oils and Aromatherapy*, an excellent introduction to the subject, English aromatherapist Valerie Ann Worwood, Ph.D., recommends adding 2 to 5 drops of essential oil to 1 teaspoon carrier oil, which is 6 to 15 drops per tablespoon, or 48 to 120 drops per ½ cup. The result is a blend that is 3 to 8 percent essential oil.

Most blends for canine application are safe and effective in concentrations of up to 10 percent essential oil. The essential oils that require the greatest dilution for use with dogs include basil, cinnamon bark, citrus (lemon, orange, grapefruit, tangerine, etc.), clove bud, eucalyptus, lemongrass, oregano, pennyroyal, peppermint, rosemary, tea tree, and thyme.

Higher concentrations are appropriate for essential oils that are gentle and well tolerated, such as fennel, best known as a digestive aid; frankincense, which eases shortness of breath, stimulates the immune system, helps heal tumors, and improves digestion; myrrh, a specific for fungal infections and other skin conditions, gingivitis, and thyroid imbalances; neroli (orange flower), recommended for sensitive skin, the respiratory system, circulation, digestion, anxiety, and depression; palmarosa (often confused with rose geranium), a circulatory stimulant that helps heal skin conditions such as hot spots and relieves stress; patchouli, an antiviral, antifungal wound healer; rose, an antiseptic, skin-healing, balancing oil; vetiver, a hormone-balancing oil traditionally used to regenerate the skin; peppermint, which has dozens of therapeutic uses, including the treatment of skin and coat, respiratory, circulatory, immune system, digestive, and nervous problems; pine, especially Scotch pine needle oil, which eases breathing, disinfects wounds, stimulates the immune system, and combats fatigue; and rose, either French or damask, which repairs the skin, improves digestion, calms the nervous system, and lifts the spirits.

ARTHRITIS MASSAGE OIL

Recommended for dogs with arthritis, this massage oil appears in Worwood's *Complete Book of Essential Oils and Aromatherapy*.

Blend 4 drops rosemary oil, 2 drops lavender oil, and 3 drops ginger oil in 1 to 2 teaspoons vegetable oil. Work well into the muscles, joints, and vertebrae.

"Don't worry about this being messy," wrote Worwood. "Your dog will soon lick much of the oil off, but by then the correct amount of essential oil will have penetrated the skin." In addition to reaching the affected tissue and bone, whatever the dog swallows will be distributed through digestion. Rosemary and ginger are warming oils that increase local blood circulation.

Diluting essential oils in water. Because essential oils do not dissolve in water, an intermediate step is needed before they can be diluted with herbal tea, aloe vera juice, water, and other fat-free liquids.

When essential oils are first dissolved in alcohol, glycerine, sulfated castor oil, soap, or any other water-soluble solvent, they disperse in water without floating to the top. Small quantities of essential oil can be added to salt with the same result, as in bath salts. Although rubbing alcohol (isopropyl alcohol) will dissolve essential oils, it has its own strong fragrance and is toxic when swallowed. For these reasons, it is not recommended for use with pets.

ESSENTIAL OIL COAT-BRUSHING TREATMENT

Recommended for dogs to repel fleas and ticks and improve coat condition.

Wrap a wire or bristle brush with several layers of cheese-cloth or a similar loosely woven absorbent fabric. The bristles should protrude about 1 inch or more, depending on the length of your dog's coat.

Mix 8 to 12 drops of insect-repelling essential oils, such as atlas cedar, pine, citronella, palmarosa, tea tree, clove, opopanax, or eucalyptus, with 2 tablespoons vodka or 1 tablespoon vegetable glycerine or sulfated castor oil.

Add 1 cup aloe vera juice or gel and 1 cup strongly brewed chamomile tea. (Use 2 cups aloe vera juice without tea for white-coated pets.)

Dip the fabric-covered brush into this mixture, then brush the dog. This treatment disinfects and conditions the coat while picking up parasites and their eggs. Thoroughly rinse the brush every few minutes, soak it again, and continue brushing. Towel-dry the dog and, if desired, complete her drying with a blow dryer.

To use this treatment for cats, substitute hydrosols and use 2 table-spoons hydrosol, ½ cup aloe vera juice, ½ cup water, and 1 cup herbal tea.

SOOTHING EAR PUFFS

This ear-cleaning formula was developed for dogs by Kristen Leigh Bell for Aromaleigh, Inc.

In a 4-ounce jar, place ½ teaspoon vegetable glycerine, 1 tablespoon vodka, 1 ounce (2 tablespoons) witch hazel hydrosol or alcohol-free witch hazel, 1 ounce aloe vera gel or juice, 1 tablespoon apple cider vinegar, 1 tablespoon Roman chamomile hydrosol, and 5 drops liquid grapefruit seed extract. Add 4 drops lavender, 6 drops bergamot, 3 drops niaouli, and 2 drops Roman chamomile essential oil.

Close the jar, shake it vigorously for 30 seconds, take
the lid off, and quickly fill the jar with cotton balls, round
cotton cosmetic pads, or paper towels cut to fit.

"I developed this product six years ago for my Golden Retriever, Dublin,"
says Bell. "I wanted something that would be easy to use, gentle, soothing,
and cleansing. The essential oils relieve itching and help prevent bacterial
and fungal infections. Refrigerating the jar keeps the product fresh and
makes this treatment cool and comfortable. You can add the same essential oils to 1 tablespoon olive oil for a soothing, infection-fighting ear oil
for use after wiping the ears."

HEALING SKIN SPRAY

Recommended for dogs with open, oozing sores, hot spots,
and wounds that won't heal.

In a glass jar containing 1 cup unrefined sea salt or
kosher salt, add ½ teaspoon (30 drops) essential oil of
chamomile, lavender, frankincense, myrrh, rose, or sandalwood,
or ½ teaspoon of any combination of these. Shake and rotate the
sealed jar to mix well. When needed, dissolve 1 tablespoon salt
in ¼ cup cool water. Spray on skin or saturate cotton and apply.

As noted on page 76, unrefined sea salt has its own healing properties. To
adapt this formula for use on cats, add 1 teaspoon unrefined sea salt or
kosher salt to ¼ cup full-strength hydrosol. Apply to cuts, wounds, burns,
abrasions, and other injuries as needed.

Diluting essential oils with fabric. Fabrics absorb essential oils and hold
their fragrance for weeks. An easy way to provide the benefits of an essential oil without applying it to your pet's skin is to treat her bedding, collar,
or scarf. The following example repels fleas, but you could as easily use an
oil that lifts depression or stimulates the immune system.

INSTANT FLEA COLLAR

Suzanne Catty recommends this easy flea collar for dogs and cats.

Place 4 drops of cedar essential oil (use atlas cedar, *Cedrus atlantica*, not the harsher Texas or Virginia cedars, *Juniperus mexicana* or *J. virginia*) on a fabric collar, piece of rope, or bandanna. Seal it in an airtight plastic bag or jar and leave overnight.

"This permeates the entire cloth," she explains. "Then just tie it around the animal's neck. It will remain effective for two to three weeks. When it needs recharging, pop it back in the bag or jar and repeat the process. Be sure to use atlas cedar for this collar, because Texas cedar is neurologically toxic to cats."

As described in my *Encyclopedia of Natural Pet Care*, the essential oils of palmarosa (often labeled rose geranium, though that is a different plant) and opopanax (the myrrh of ancient Egypt) are effective tick repellents. According to Catty, atlas cedar repels ticks and can be blended with these oils to improve their performance. To make a tick-repelling collar, follow the directions above using 1 to 2 drops each of opopanax, palmarosa, and atlas cedar.

Diluting essential oils in powders. Another way to make essential oils safe for external application is to dilute them in powders. Baking soda, which has its own deodorizing properties, is widely used, but you can substitute rice flour, cornstarch, or any other nontoxic powder. If using clay, use a mild one that won't dry the skin excessively, or add a small amount to one of the other recommended powders.

FLEA POWDER

Recommended for use on dogs and cats. This formula was developed by Suzanne Catty.

Combine 3 parts atlas cedar, 2 parts pine, and 1 part niaouli or tea tree oil. Both niaouli and tea tree are Australian

Melaleuca species, and they have similar disinfecting properties. Use 12 to 15 drops of this essential oil blend per cup of
baking soda, or use a blend of baking soda and rice flour. Stir
or shake to mix well.

"If you have fleas," says Catty, "put this powder on your pets and, after
vacuuming, sprinkle it on furniture, carpets, floors, curtains, animal bedding, and everywhere fleas might hide. Let the powder stand for 30 to 60
minutes, then vacuum again. Do this once a week and you will be flea-free
forever." To make a tick-repelling powder, add palmarosa or opopanax
essential oil to the formula, as described above.

Powders are a safe, gentle way to apply other essential oils to dogs
and cats. Patricia Whitaker at Scents of Smell developed a lavender pet
powder using a blend of lavender, ylang ylang, bergamot, and melissa oils.
"I developed this formula for anxiety," she explains, "such as when
stressed owners are separated from their stressed pets for long periods.
Sprinkle it wherever you and your pet spend time, and it will help both of
you relax. When I got my dog Cookie from the pound, I put it on a blan-
ket for her ride home. I've since found that the product is effective on
smelly bedding and carpeting."

To experiment with this method, follow the flea powder recipe
above and substitute other essential oils.

Tea tree oil. Tea tree oil is used to treat skin lesions, insect bites, rashes,
burns, abscesses, cuts, abrasions, infected wounds, and fungal infections.
Like eucalyptus oil, tea tree oil is a specific for the respiratory system as
well as an all-purpose disinfectant. Australian and British research conducted in the 1930s showed that a 15 percent tea tree oil solution is as
effective as the full-strength oil in killing yeast cells, mold, bacteria, and
viruses. More recent laboratory tests have shown that concentrations as low
as 1 percent are effective against streptococcus and other gram-positive
bacteria, *E. coli* and other gram-negative bacteria, and several fungi.

Because pets find its turpentine taste unpleasant, some holistic pet guides recommend the application of tea tree oil to body parts that an animal chews or licks incessantly, such as the leg or tail. Such guides usually list full-strength tea tree oil as appropriate for use on insect bites, burns, infected wounds, cuts, ringworm, and other fungal infections. However, temporary paralysis caused by the use of undiluted tea tree oil has been reported to the National Animal Poison Control Center following such use on dogs and cats. Symptoms, which occurred within two to eight hours of application, included depression, weakness, incoordination, and muscle tremors. The reaction disappeared within three to four days. A 10 percent solution of tea tree oil is unlikely to cause adverse side effects in dogs if used sparingly.

10 PERCENT TEA TREE OIL SOLUTION

Use this procedure to dilute any essential oil in a carrier oil. Recommended for dogs with skin conditions, infected wounds, burns, pustules, and ringworm.

Add 1 tablespoon full-strength tea tree oil to ½ cup carrier oil. Stir to mix well. Pour into an amber-glass bottle and label. Attach a rubber eyedropper to the bottle with a rubber band for convenient application. Do not use a rubber eyedropper cap for long-term storage because essential oils dissolve rubber.

Use this oil wherever you want to prevent the solution from being washed or rinsed away. This diluted oil can be added to ear oils used to treat bacterial infections of the ear, or it can be applied to the skin of a dog who is going swimming. Keep this and all tea tree oil products away from the eyes.

7 PERCENT TEA TREE OIL SOLUTION

Use this procedure to dilute any essential oil in water, tea, aloe vera gel, or other nonfat liquids. Recommended for disinfecting household surfaces and for topical use on dogs.

Add 1 tablespoon full-strength tea tree oil to 2 ounces (4 tablespoons) vodka, other grain alcohol, vegetable glycerine, or sulfated castor oil. Shake or stir well and let stand for 10 seconds. If a film of oil floats to the top, add more liquid and shake again. When no oil floats to the surface, pour the solution into a measuring cup and add enough aloe vera juice or gel, herbal tea such as comfrey or calendula, pure water, or any combination of aloe, tea, and water to fill the cup to the 6-ounce or ¾-cup mark. At that point, your solution will be approximately 7 percent tea tree oil.

This same procedure works with any essential oil, not just tea tree. Water-soluble solutions of essential oils are the foundation of many aromatherapy products, from soaks and lotions to air sprays. If small amounts of oil separate later, simply shake the product before using.

This 7 percent tea tree oil solution can be sprayed on kitchen and bathroom surfaces, into air ducts or air-conditioning units, and on telephone receivers and mildewed shower walls. It can be added to laundry wash water or simply sprayed into the air. Groomers, animal shelter workers, trainers, and boarding kennel operators can guard against infectious diseases such as kennel cough with this spray.

Tea tree oil should not be used every day on every surface, for immunologists report that regular exposure may cause bacteria, viruses, and other agents of infection to become resistant to the oil's effects. Instead of relying on a single disinfecting agent, use several in rotation, such as dilute solutions of the essential oils of myrrh, pine, cloves, juniper berries, oregano, and thyme, teas brewed from sage and chaparral, and dilute solutions of liquid grapefruit seed extract.

DEODORANT AIR SPRAY

Recommended for the removal of pet odors and as an
all-purpose air freshener.

Combine 6 parts lavendin (a lavender hybrid), 3 parts
terebinth, 2 parts lemon, and 1 part mint essential oils.

Use full-strength in a diffuser or dilute with vodka,
glycerine, or sulfated castor oil and water for use in a
plastic spray bottle; then spray the air, avoiding pets
and their food.

According to Nelly Grosjean, this blend, manufactured in France under the
brand name Freshtonic, satisfies the greatest number of users and is not
disliked by cats. Its strong, fresh smell and antiseptic action help eliminate
pet odors.

Adding essential oils to food. Essential oils can be added to food in small
amounts to improve digestion, fight parasites, stimulate kidney function,
improve vitality, lift the spirits, relieve pain, enhance sleep, help an anxious
pet relax, improve immune function, and speed the healing of wounds.
Their internal use is controversial, with some schools of aromatherapy
warning that essential oils should never be swallowed by pets or people.
However, essential oils are used throughout the food and beverage industry as natural flavorings, and in France and Germany essential oils are routinely taken by mouth.

Cats lack the liver enzymes that help canines and humans detoxify
drugs, and only a few aromatherapists recommend that essential oils be
added to their food. Hydrosols are much safer for use with cats.

Dogs seem to tolerate essential oils well, but they should be introduced in small quantities. Give 1 drop essential oil per 45 to 50 pounds of
body weight per dose. To divide 1 drop for smaller dogs, mix it into a small
amount of food and divide the food, or dilute a measured number of drops
in a larger quantity of edible oil or powdered herbs. For example, 1 drop

of essential oil in 1 teaspoon olive oil or powdered wheat grass can be divided into four ¼-teaspoon or eight ⅛-teaspoon servings.

Treat acute conditions for three to seven days, giving 1 dose two to three times daily. For preventive or post-crisis use, give 1 dose per day for one to three weeks.

Not all essential oils are safe for internal use, and some that are should not be used during pregnancy. In general, it is best to substitute hydrosols for use with young puppies, pregnant dogs, dogs in frail health, seizure-prone dogs, and cats of all ages.

To give hydrosols internally, Suzanne Catty recommends adding ¼ teaspoon hydrosol per cup to water for drinking or tea brewing. "Dogs and cats tolerate carrot seed hydrosol exceptionally well," she says, "and they also like the taste of balsam fir and black spruce, both of which are immune system boosters."

Full-strength hydrosols can be added to food at 1 drop per pound of body weight per day, which is ½ teaspoon for a 30-pound dog and 1 tea-spoon for a 60-pound dog. "For a health maintenance regime, this works well," says Catty. "You can treat chronic conditions with 2 drops per pound on a three-weeks-on, one-week-off cycle. This way the body has a week to assimilate the changes and healing process; then the treatment can be reevaluated and adjusted as necessary. For acute conditions, give 2 drops per pound per day." With their sensitive noses, dogs and cats may not want to drink water to which hydrosols have been added, but they usually accept hydrosols in food.

SWEET BREATH BLEND

Recommended for dogs.

Combine equal parts caraway, chamomile, coriander, and lavender essential oils. Add 1 drop to food daily for small dogs, 2 drops for large dogs, and 3 drops for giant breeds.

This blend can be used to improve digestion as well as deodorize the animal from within. For cats, substitute hydrosols, adding 5 to 10 drops per serving.

Essential oil tooth and gum care. "For all tooth and gum problems," says Catty, "whether human, canine, or feline, the hydrosol of choice is helichrysum, the Italian immortelle. Because it has the ability to regenerate cells, it helps repair receding gums, swelling, bleeding, and infection. For animals with gum problems, I also use balsam fir, which is a good general tonic and immune booster."

To use a hydrosol for these conditions, Catty suggests pouring a small amount in a glass, dipping your finger or a feline toothbrush, and gently rubbing it along your pet's teeth and gums. Alternatively, use a small spray bottle to spray it directly into the animal's mouth.

"Cats won't like it much," she warns, "but in addition to adding hydrosols to food, this is the best way to treat an infection."

If the underlying cause is digestive, she recommends carrot seed or peppermint hydrosol. If an abscess is draining, bay laurel (bay leaf) hydrosol combined with helichrysum hydrosol supports the lymph system as it removes infection. Where bleeding is a factor, yarrow hydrosol is effective.

"Choose one or two hydrosols," she suggests, "and apply them to the affected area, add them to food, and put them in your pet's drinking water."

Although Catty does not recommend using essential oils on cats, she makes an exception for abscessed teeth. "For a cat with an abscess," she says, "I would add 1 drop clove oil to 2 drops olive oil and use a cotton swab to paint it directly on the abscess. Even better would be 1 drop clove and 1 drop palmarosa in 4 drops olive oil. Palmarosa is antifungal, antibacterial, antiviral, antiseptic, immune-boosting, and extremely gentle. It cools the mouth and is a perfect partner to clove oil, which acts as a topical anesthetic."

Preventing and Treating Contagious Diseases

With a natural diet in place, supplements in the cupboard, herbs on hand, and essential oils in the medicine cabinet, you are well equipped to prevent and treat the most common canine and feline conditions.

Contagious diseases worry all pet owners. It is easier to prevent an illness than to treat one, but as holistic veterinarians are quick to point out, animals fed a natural diet tend to have shorter, less severe cases of common illnesses than average pets.

Using Herbs to Boost Immunity

The first rule of healthy living is to be a poor host to disease. Strengthening immunity with herbs and nutritional supplements enhances the body's complex systems of self-defense.

Two families of herbs used on a regular basis build immunity by strengthening the entire system. These are tonic herbs, which nourish the whole body, and adaptogen herbs, which restore balance to any part of the body that is underactive or overactive. Dandelion is one of the best-known tonic herbs; it has a beneficial effect on the digestion, kidneys, urinary tract, liver, skin, and circulation. Ginseng is the best-known adaptogen herb, famous for restoring vitality and improving overall health by correcting imbalances. Both tonic and adaptogen herbs are safe for long-term daily use; in fact, their success depends on it.

The daily use of tonic and adaptogen herbs such as aloe vera, ashwagandha, astragalus, bupleurum, cinnamon, fo-ti, ginseng, medicinal mushrooms (cordyceps, maitake, reishi, shiitake, and others), microalgae (chlorella, spirulina, and other one-celled plants), schisandra, Siberian ginseng, turmeric and/or wheatgrass, and other cereal grasses will help your pet resist disease.

Echinacea is promoted as an immune-boosting herb, and while it deserves that reputation, there is disagreement in herbal circles about its best use. Some believe echinacea should be reserved until needed, then given immediately after exposure to an active illness or at the first sign of infection, using large amounts (double or triple the usual dosages) for short periods (less than two weeks). Others have found that giving echinacea on a regular basis so stimulates the immune system that animals resist infections they would normally contract.

To take advantage of both approaches, add small amounts of echinacea to your pet's food every few days, and when she is exposed to kennel cough, a respiratory infection, or any communicable disease, or the minute she comes down with something, use echinacea in large amounts. Used swiftly and in frequent doses, such as every hour, echinacea can cure a viral or bacterial infection overnight.

Marina Zacharias reviewed echinacea's scientific literature in the February/March 1999 edition of her *Natural Rearing Newsletter*. Citing extensive German studies, Zacharias refuted the "do not use for more than ten days at a time" warning commonly applied to this herb. She recommends therapeutic doses of echinacea for both long and short periods for pets.

Supporting the Lymph System

The lymph system is often overlooked in discussions of this kind, but it is a key component of the immune system. Lymph circulates in its own channels, collecting dead cells and other debris for removal from the body. Three important ways to stimulate the circulation of lymph are active exercise, deep breathing, and brushing. Running, jumping, climbing, rolling over, and chasing toys are important activities for dogs and cats, especially when they stimulate deep breathing. In addition to playing with your pet and taking your dog for hikes and swims, devote a few minutes each day to vigorous brushing. Use a natural-bristle brush and work up from the feet to the trunk, down the spine, and around the neck and chest. This brushing has nothing to do with grooming; its purpose is to stimulate the skin and lymph circulation. The herb cleavers, also known as clinging bedstraw, is a specific for the lymph, as are the essential oils and hydrosols of immortelle (*Helichrysum* species) and lemon.

Reduce Exposure to Harmful Pathogens

In addition to strengthening your pet's immune system to make him a poor host to pathogens, you can reduce his exposure to them. Give filtered or bottled spring water, feed organically raised foods whenever possible, and practice good hygiene. Public health officials are concerned about the growing use of antibacterial soaps and topical disinfectants on hands and in kitchens because these products actually contribute to the creation of supergerms, just as the indiscriminate use of antibiotics creates drug-resistant bacteria. Regular soap and hot water disinfects hands and kitchen surfaces effectively.

If it is necessary to use a more powerful disinfectant, such as when a family member or visitor is ill with a contagious disease or when a visitor's pet is ill, even if the animal does not come into your house, herbs and essential oils can be used as topical disinfectants (see page 187). It is a good idea to switch from one to another, just as it's a good idea to use different medicinal herbs in rotation.

Herbal Immunization

Juliette de Bairacli Levy has used no vaccines, antibiotics, or other drugs on her animals for more than fifty years, and neither have adherents of her Natural Rearing philosophy. In *The Complete Herbal Handbook for the Dog and Cat*, she describes an "intensive herbal immunization" that can be used for pets exposed to active infections. The treatment is a half-day or one-day fast (water only) with a laxative that night followed by a dose of herbal antiseptic tablets (see Resources), which contain garlic, rue, sage, thyme, eucalyptus, wormwood, and vegetable charcoal. Alternatively, combine minced garlic with enough whole-wheat flour and honey to make a dough, divide the mixture into small pills, and add 1 drop of eucalyptus essential oil to each. Give 1 tablet or pill per 10 pounds of body weight for several days. As a general preventive, Levy recommends giving antiseptic herbs to dogs just before attending shows or visiting public parks.

Using herbal immunization, Levy has protected unvaccinated dogs, cats, sheep, cattle, and other animals exposed to epidemics. In one case, she saved 2,000 pedigree Swaledale sheep in the English Pennine mountains by dosing them heavily while the sheep in an adjacent field succumbed to a streptococcal infection that caused paralysis and blindness. None of the sheep treated with herbs became ill.

Here is a review of natural immunizations that can help your pet resist or recover from contagious diseases.

- Fast the animal by withholding food for ½ to 1 day if exposed to an illness; if the animal has a fever, withhold food until the fever breaks. See the fasting safeguards on page 97.
- Give the animal several tablets or capsules of food-source vitamin C throughout the day. Crush or grind tablets or use a powdered or liquid supplement for easy assimilation. If a food-source supplement isn't available, use calcium ascorbate (such as Ester C) with bioflavonoids, 500 milligrams per 10 pounds of body weight. See page 67.
- In addition, give any of the following per day in divided doses. These recommendations are safe for short-term use and should be started as quickly as possible, at the first sign of infection or as soon as the animal is exposed to a contagious illness.

  Choose one:

  - 1 herbal antiseptic tablet or garlic-eucalyptus pill per 10 pounds of body weight as described above.
  - 1 capsule of powdered grapefruit seed extract per 10 to 25 pounds of body weight, or 1½ drops of liquid grapefruit seed extract per pound.
  - 1 or 2 drops of propolis tincture per pound of body weight, or 250 milligrams powdered propolis from capsules per 5 to 7 pounds.

- 1 garlic extract capsule (Khryolic or a similar brand) per 10 pounds of body weight, ¼ teaspoon garlic tincture per 10 pounds, or ⅛ teaspoon finely chopped, minced, or pureed garlic per 10 pounds.
- 1 drop of echinacea tincture per pound of body weight, 1 tablespoon of medicinal-strength echinacea tea per 10 pounds, or 3 capsules of powdered echinacea per 10 pounds.
- 1 to 3 drops ryegrass extract (Oralmat); see page 82.
- Adapt the label directions of any infection-fighting herb or supplement, such as olive leaf extract, noni, astragalus, colostrum, or lactoferrin, to your pet's weight.

Do not feed an herb or supplement that should be taken with meals to a fasting animal. Check labels carefully.

The above are one-day dosages that should be divided into three or more servings during the day. Use any of the above alone, or alternate from one to another. Continue these dosages for three days as a preventive or up to ten days to treat an active infection.

The only appropriate foods for a fasting animal are raw, unpasteurized honey or a mixture of slippery elm bark and water (see page 158), either of which can be mixed with supplements such as vitamin C, herbal powders, crushed tablets, whole capsules or their contents, tinctures, or strongly brewed herbal tea. See page 98 for the nutrients needed for effective detoxification during fasting. Shape refrigerated honey into balls, feed room-temperature honey or slippery elm syrup from a spoon, or dilute honey with water or herb tea and gently pour it into your pet's mouth or cheek pouch. Encourage your fasting pet to drink water, and make clean water (add Willard Water extract and a pinch of unrefined sea salt) available at all times.

Essential oil immunization. In France, where essential oils are taken internally as medicines, physicians who practice aromatherapy take a culture from the infected patient and cultivate it in order to test the effect of individual essential oils on the infection. The oils that most successfully inhibit the culture's growth are combined in a prescription to be used until the infection subsides.

Some of the most widely prescribed all-purpose oils are combined in formulas that are sold to prevent infections before they spread. In *Veterinary Aromatherapy*, Nelly Grosjean describes how to make such a blend for pets. Combine equal parts of the essential oils of thyme, cinnamon, coriander, clove, nutmeg, pine, and ylang ylang, then mix this blend with an equal quantity of the essential oil of wild marjoram (*Origanum vulgare*). Dose the exposed or infected animal 3 times daily with 1 drop of the mixture per 20 pounds of body weight.

This aromatic blend helps prevent and treat bacterial, viral, and other infectious diseases. Its topical use in sprays and massage oils enhances mental alertness, physical equilibrium, memory, sexual drive, and cellular vitality.

In addition to giving the animal the essential oils described above, combine the following essential oils for continuous use in an aromatic diffuser: 8 parts lavender, 4 parts eucalyptus; 2 parts each thyme, wild marjoram, and rosemary; and 1 part each mint and cinnamon. If you define 1 part as ⅛ teaspoon, the result will be 2½ teaspoons of the blend. If you don't have a diffuser, combine the mixture with 2 tablespoons vodka or other 80-proof grain alcohol and add it to ½ cup of water in a small spray bottle. Every 15 minutes, or whenever you think of it, spray the air in the room around your pet.

The spread of airborne viruses and bacteria can be greatly reduced by spraying the air, kennel surfaces, and other areas with solutions of grapefruit seed extract, tea tree oil, or the essential oils of other antiseptic herbs.

Herbal Replacements for Topical Antibiotics

Eye infections, burns, infected cuts, abrasions, leg ulcers, and other wounds are often treated with antibiotic ointments. These drugs have the same limitations as antibiotics that are ingested or injected; as bacteria adapt and become drug-resistant, topical antibiotics lose their effectiveness, and some animals are allergic to prescription antibiotics. Wounds that refuse to heal despite weeks of treatment with antibiotic ointments may respond overnight to medicinal herbs.

One of the fastest and most effective ways to clear infection from a tender, swollen, oozing sore is with a poultice made of comfrey, plantain, or wheat grass (see page 165). Even a bruised cabbage leaf can be used for this purpose with good results.

Many essential oils are antiseptic; in fact, more than sixty popular essential oils kill bacteria on contact. The essential oils with the greatest disinfecting properties are those that are antiviral and antifungal as well, such as cinnamon, cloves, eucalyptus, lavender, onion, oregano, sandalwood, tea tree, and thyme. All of these essential oils can be diluted for topical use on dogs as described on pages 186–187. Their hydrosols can be used on both dogs and cats.

Bee propolis (see page 80) is an excellent topical disinfectant and natural antibiotic. Liquid propolis can be applied to cuts, wounds, burns, scratches, and other injuries with an eyedropper, or it can be mixed with small amounts of aloe vera gel to treat larger areas.

Propolis derives its antiseptic properties from the sap of poplar tree buds and pitch, the resinous sap of coniferous trees. A folk remedy for centuries, pitch has antibacterial, antiviral, and antifungal properties. It has been used by veterinarians and physicians to treat skin infections, black widow and brown recluse spider bites, flea and tick bites, wasp and bee stings, ear infections, gum infections, poison oak and ivy rashes, ringworm, staph infections, and burns and scalds. Its only adverse side effect is that it is highly flammable and should not be used around fire or flame. It is also sticky.

If coniferous trees on your property exude resin from injuries to the bark or in resin-filled blisters that can be punctured and pressed, collect this fragrant, healing ingredient for your pet's first-aid kit. The North American Tree Resin Company (NATR; see Resources) is the leading retail source of undiluted tree resin and products made from the pitch of Pacific Coast Douglas fir, yellow pine, and other coniferous trees. Add liquid pitch to any salve recipe in any proportion, mix full-strength pitch with a small amount of olive oil, apply liquid pitch full-strength to injuries, or cover solid pitch with alcohol to make a disinfecting tincture for external use. Pitch can be applied diluted or full-strength to any cut, burn, abrasion, infected wound, or injury (avoid the eyes and mucous membranes).

To sweeten your dog's breath, combine ⅛ teaspoon pitch with 8 drops mastic or myrrh essential oil and 8 drops lavender essential oil in 1 teaspoon almond oil or a similar carrier oil. Apply a small amount to your dog's toothbrush or to a gauze pad wrapped around your finger. Gently massage the teeth and gums.

Traditional herbal medicine makes extensive use of tree resins. The most famous are myrrh and frankincense, which have been treasured for millennia for their fragrance as well as their antiseptic applications. Another famous resin is mastic, which has recently been shown to cure human stomach ulcers by destroying *Helicobacter pylori* bacteria and which may have a similarly beneficial effect on the digestive tracts of animals. Mastic is best known as a therapy for gum disease (see tooth powder recipe on pages 166–167) and as a breath sweetener (see above). Mastic essential oil or mastic gum can be added to a pet's food to repair damage to gastric mucosa, protect tissue against damage from irritants, and destroy harmful bacteria, including those associated with food poisoning.

DISINFECTING LIQUID SALVE

Recommended for dogs and cats with infected wounds, puncture wounds, hot spots, ringworm, cuts, burns, and other injuries.

Combine ¼ cup castor oil, 1 tablespoon liquid pitch, 1 tablespoon neem seed oil, and 1 teaspoon lavender essential oil.

This sticky salve adheres to skin and fur, so apply
carefully with an eyedropper or similar applicator. Avoid
the eyes. An all-purpose first-aid therapy, this combination is
highly effective. Castor oil is deeply penetrating, and the other
ingredients are highly antiseptic and stimulate healing. If
desired, this mixture can be diluted with an equal amount
of comfrey-infused olive oil (see page 169).

Eye care. Several herbs have a special affinity for the eyes and help clear
eye infections. Goldenseal tea, also called eye balm, is a traditional eye
wash. Simmer 1 teaspoon goldenseal root (or 1 teabag) in 2 cups water for
5 minutes and let stand until cool. Add 2 drops liquid grapefruit seed
extract plus ½ teaspoon unrefined sea salt or boric acid powder or both.
Strain the liquid through fabric or filter paper. Warm the solution to body
temperature and apply it to your pet's eyes with an eyedropper (tilt the
head back and apply drops in the outside corner), spray it from a spray
bottle, or saturate cotton or gauze and hold it over your pet's closed eyes
as long as possible. Because goldenseal tea is dark yellow in color, it may
stain white fur.

For pets with a chronic eye discharge, alternate an eyewash made
from goldenseal tea and boric acid with one made from an eyebright infusion (steeped tea) and salt, changing from one to the other every two or
three days. Alternating between an acid and alkaline wash and between
these two eye-friendly herbs will help clear any chronic discharge. For pets
with white fur, alternate between eyebright tea with boric acid and eyebright tea without it.

Neem tea is a specific for conjunctivitis and other eye infections.
Willard Water is another eye-friendly ingredient; applied by itself, it improves eye health, and in solution with herbs it improves their effectiveness. Willard Water extract can be added to the water used to make any eyewash. Castor oil is a specific for eye infections, styes, and conjunctivitis. It
can be applied full-strength with an eyedropper.

Wound healing. Unrefined sea salt, with its abundant trace minerals, is an effective skin healer. A female German Shepherd Dog in Samantha's obedience class suffered from a sore that wouldn't heal despite repeated trips to the veterinarian. When her owner applied a solution of unrefined sea salt and water, the sore improved the same day and healed within a week. Combining sea salt with healing herbs is an excellent way to enhance skin cell repair.

ELECTROLYTE HERBAL SPRAY

Recommended for dogs and cats with any skin disorder. This recipe uses dried herbs; if using fresh herbs, double or triple the quantity of each herb.

In a covered pan, combine 2 tablespoons each chopped burdock root, comfrey root, horsetail, and juniper berries in 2 quarts (8 cups) water. Bring to a boil, then gently simmer for 15 to 20 minutes. Remove from heat. Add 2 tablespoons each chamomile blossoms, comfrey leaf, calendula blossoms, lavender blossoms, and St. John's wort blossoms. If all of these ingredients are not available, use whichever ones you have for a total of about 1 cup dried herbs. Stir these into the tea, replace the cover, and let stand until cool. Strain the tea through a cloth and press the residue to release as much liquid as possible. You will have about 6 cups of tea.

Add 1 cup aloe vera juice or gel, ½ cup unrefined sea salt, and 2 tablespoons liquid grapefruit seed extract to the strained tea. If available, add 2 tablespoons liquid pitch or tree resin. All of the herbs in this formula have significant skin-healing properties, and the unrefined sea salt provides trace elements that speed wound healing and repair the skin. The grapefruit seed extract and pitch fight infection and act as natural preservatives.

Although the salt, grapefruit seed extract, and pitch will retard spoilage, keep this solution refrigerated for long-term storage. Use a plant mister or other spray bottle to apply the tea to any cut, wound, burn, abrasion, bite, scratch, infection, or other injury, spraying it on the affected area several times per day. Alternatively, soak a piece of gauze or cotton and apply it as a compress, or simply pour the solution onto the injury as a wash or rinse. Even wounds that have not responded to conventional treatment heal rapidly when treated with this combination of skin-repairing nutrients.

MEDICATED HONEY FORMULA

Recommended for all skin injuries, especially scalds and burns. Honey by itself is a highly effective burn treatment because it seals the skin, protects it from exposure to oxygen, eliminates the need for frequent bandage changes, and prevents healing skin from adhering to gauze or fabric.

Buy a plastic squeeze bottle of honey. Don't use raw honey for this purpose as it tends to crystallize, forming sharp points that are painful to burned or injured skin. Buy clear, pasteurized, filtered honey, or warm raw honey until it is hot to the touch and no longer raw, then strain it through cheese-cloth and let it cool. To 1 cup of room-temperature honey, add ½ teaspoon full-strength tea tree oil, 1 teaspoon liquid grape-fruit seed extract, 1 teaspoon essential oil of lavender, and, if available, 1 tablespoon neem seed oil or liquid pitch.

Most dogs and cats dislike the bitter taste of grapefruit seed extract and the turpentine fragrance of tea tree oil, but if they lick off small amounts, this medicated honey won't hurt them. Label the container "Medicated Honey for Burns and Wounds. External Use." Apply to any infected area.

When Antibiotics Are Necessary

Veterinarians differ as to when antibiotics are necessary, but the odds are that a pet in your household has taken these prescription drugs more than once.

Although not always obvious, the side effects of antibiotics can be serious. Pets as well as people die from allergic reactions. Antibiotics have been blamed for birth defects in kittens and puppies conceived while either parent was taking the drug or born to mothers who were treated while pregnant. Because they disrupt an animal's intestinal flora by destroying beneficial as well as harmful bacteria, antibiotic treatment is often followed by bouts of indigestion, systemic yeast infections, thrush, ear infections, and other problems caused by the opportunistic growth of bacteria no longer held in check by natural defenses.

Another inconvenient side effect is the disruption of scent detection in hunting, tracking, and search and rescue dogs. Some experts theorize that by destroying the beneficial bacteria in a dog's nose, antibiotics confuse the animal's ability to detect and process the minute information that makes his sense of smell 300 million times more acute than our own. This temporary disability is often apparent during the second week of antibiotic treatment and up to two weeks after treatment stops. If you engage in activities that depend on your dog's good nose, the use of natural infection fighters will prevent this side effect.

No one says that antibiotics should never be used for any patient under any circumstances, for antibiotics can and do save lives, but holistic veterinarians criticize their casual use, especially when their side effects outweigh their benefits and when natural therapies are equally or more effective.

Your pet is most likely to benefit from antibiotics when taking them for a short course (typically seven to fourteen days) for a serious condition such as a paralyzing attack of Lyme disease, a dental abscess that is poisoning the entire body, or a life-threatening bladder infection. Fewer benefits come from their long-term use for chronic or recurring infections, and antibiotics offer no protection against viruses. There is no justification for dosing dogs and cats with antibiotics "just in case" the drugs might prevent a problem that the veterinarian hasn't diagnosed.

Holistic veterinarians who prescribe antibiotics often give large amounts of vitamin C at the same time, sometimes double or triple the animal's normal daily dose, to help counteract their side effects.

Because antibiotics disrupt your pet's intestinal balance, there is no point in trying to correct this imbalance until after the treatment. The day antibiotic treatment ends, begin dosing your pet with large quantities of acidophilus supplements, freshly prepared yogurt or kefir, lactic acid fermented vegetables, and other foods that contain or feed beneficial bacteria. Garlic taken the week after therapy ends helps cleanse the intestinal tract and make it more hospitable to the friendly bacteria introduced by acidophilus and other supplements. In addition, fresh cleavers and dandelion act as tonics for the spleen and lymph, helping restore normal function to the entire system. Add either or both to your pet's food as available.

Veterinary homeopaths rarely recommend antibiotics. Consult an expert before treating any serious condition to be sure you're using the correct preparation. If you pet has taken antibiotics in the past, consult a veterinary homeopath for post-treatment guidelines.

Herbal Support for Detoxification

Of the many bodily functions that promote and maintain good health, one of the most important is detoxification. Without the right foods, the body's filters can't work efficiently. Providing a well-balanced, biologically appropriate raw diet is essential for kidney and liver health.

That said, several herbs and natural products enhance detoxification by providing nutritional support for the liver and kidneys, stimulating the urinary and intestinal tracts for more efficient elimination, binding with toxins to remove them from the body, or protecting the entire system with a gentle cleansing and toning action. In addition to providing the nutrients described on pages 94–98, give your pet one or more of the following herbs to prevent the symptoms of too-rapid detoxification during fasting, after an illness or conventional medical treatment, or while changing from commercial pet food to a natural diet.

Milk Thistle Seed

One of the most important liver tonic herbs is milk thistle seed. Successfully used in Europe for the treatment of mushroom poisoning, milk thistle seed protects and regenerates the liver even in cases of hepatitis, exposure to environmental toxins, and damage caused by pharmaceutical drugs. Milk thistle seeds can be ground and added to food, brewed as a tea infusion, powdered and placed in capsules, or tinctured with alcohol, vegetable glycerine, or cider vinegar. This is an excellent companion remedy for any animal receiving comfrey for an injury that involves broken bones, for milk thistle seed protects the liver from the pyrrolizidine alkaloids in untreated comfrey.

Doses of ¼ teaspoon ground seeds or 1 dropperful of tincture per 10 to 15 pounds of body weight are commonly prescribed. Because milk thistle seed is nontoxic, therapeutic doses can be higher. Most dogs and cats enjoy the taste, making it easy to administer in food or water.

Aloe Vera

Aloe vera helps remove toxins from the system while soothing the digestive tract. Daily doses protect the system from a variety of harmful compounds. During times of rapid detoxification, double the dosage. See pages 78–79 and 108 for more information.

Herbal Melange

A dark, mudlike concentrate from Austrian peat moors that contains traces of hundreds of different plant species, Herbal Melange is a traditional folk remedy with a worldwide following. Extensive research in Europe has shown that it stimulates digestion and the absorption of nutrients, absorbs gas, binds acid, lowers alcohol levels, reduces cholesterol, repels parasites, removes harmful bacteria, and detoxifies the entire gastrointestinal system.

Herbal Melange (see Resources) is an effective first-aid treatment for any animal that has been exposed to something toxic. As a support therapy for detoxification, it is unexcelled. Add small amounts to drinking water, gradually increasing the amount as your pet grows accustomed to the taste.

Essiac Tea

Essiac tea, best known as a cancer therapy, contains sheep sorrel, a wild perennial relative of garden sorrel and a blood tonic; burdock root, a well-known blood purifier and kidney cleanser; slippery elm bark, a demulcent, nutritive, tonic herb; and Turkey rhubarb root, a liver tonic, appetite stimulant, headache reliever, and digestive aid. Holistic veterinarians recommend Essiac tea in the treatment of tumors, thyroid disorders, and skin conditions, and as a general health tonic. Some do not recommend its use by humans with kidney disease or arthritis because of the arthritis-aggravating oxalic acid in sheep sorrel and Turkey rhubarb root. The blend has nonetheless helped dogs and cats with these same disorders. Turkey rhubarb root is not recommended for pregnant animals.

Veterinarian Beverly Cappel often recommends Essiac tea as a support therapy. "I use it because it flushes the system," she explains. "Some reports say that it kills cancer. It does not kill cancer, it just cleans the body out. You're opening up the kidneys and the liver, you're helping to purify the blood, and you're soothing the gastrointestinal tract. It just flushes toxins and makes the body healthier so that it can fight cancer and many other illnesses."

Essiac can be purchased as a brewed tea in bottles or made at home from dry herbs. The recommended dosage is about 1 teaspoon per 10 pounds of body weight. Cats receive ½ to 1 teaspoon daily, dogs up to 30 pounds receive 1 tablespoon, and larger dogs receive 1 tablespoon for every 30 pounds of body weight. Because Essiac is best administered on an empty stomach half an hour before meals, it is more difficult to administer to dogs and cats than preparations that can be combined with food. However, small amounts in drinking water can be gradually increased, or the tea can be given by spoon or squeeze bottle.

Bupleurum

The Chinese herb bupleurum, sold as a tea and in small tablets in preparations such as Minor Bupleurum Formula, has been reported by Western physicians to be exceptionally effective in the treatment of hepatitis, liver cancer, and other diseases of the liver. Bupleurum preparations are sold in herb shops and health food stores that carry Chinese herbs, in Chinese markets, and by mail order. Give between 1 and 2 tablespoons tea or 1 tablet per 10 pounds of body weight per day as a liver support therapy.

Medicinal Mushrooms

Maitake, reishi, shiitake, and other medicinal mushrooms have received much publicity in recent years for their immune system–stimulating properties. Increasingly popular with holistic veterinarians, combination and single-mushroom extracts are used as support therapies in the treatment of dogs, cats, and other animals with many serious illnesses. Any combination can be given with food or between meals to support efficient detoxification. Medicinal mushrooms enhance liver health and are recommended for the prevention and treatment of all liver diseases, including hepatitis.

Modified arabinoxylane (MGN-3) is a supplement made from rice bran that has been enzymatically treated with medicinal mushroom extracts. Published clinical studies indicate that MGN-3 increases natural killer (NK) cell activity and enhances immune system function, making it a promising cancer therapy and treatment for other serious illnesses.

Citrus Pectin

Like apple pectin, best known as a jelly ingredient, pectin from grapefruit and other citrus fruits is a mucilagenous, water-soluble substance that attracts and holds liquid, swelling to form a viscous, glutinous mass. The pectin's mucilage coats mucous membranes and protects them from irritation while its fiber and bulk soften bowel contents, improving elimination.

Recent clinical studies indicate that modified citrus pectin is absorbed into the bloodstream, where it attaches to unhealthy or undesirable cells, helping to remove them from the body. Any type of pectin can be added in small amounts to a pet's wet dinner or simply mixed with water on fast days to support detoxification.

Clay and Activated Charcoal

Clay is another detoxification aid that absorbs and removes toxins from the body. Because clay may bind with essential minerals and remove them as well, it is not recommended for daily use but rather for periods of fasting or rapid detoxification. Clay helps alleviate diarrhea by "gluing" fecal matter together.

Use green bentonite or montmorillonite clay powder sold for cosmetic purposes, liquid bentonite clay sold for intestinal cleansing, or Kaopectate, which contains clay and pectin. If using clay powder or a very thick liquid, mix it with enough water to make it easy to pour, and let it stand 5 to 10 minutes to be sure it's fully hydrated. Add more water as needed to maintain a liquid consistency. Give about ½ teaspoon of liquid clay or 1 teaspoon Kaopectate per 10 pounds of body weight and repeat the dose every four hours for one or two days. Give plenty of water and other fluids at the same time. Alternatively, mix a teaspoon of clay with the water in your pet's bowl. The clay will settle to the bottom, but the water will still have a therapeutic effect.

Powdered charcoal is an effective first-aid treatment for poisoning. Like clay, charcoal is best used during rapid detoxification or on fast days.

Mix powdered activated charcoal with an equal quantity of slippery elm bark powder or pectin, and add enough water to form a liquid. Give 1 to 2 teaspoons between meals to animals weighing less than 25 pounds and 2 to 3 teaspoons to dogs weighing more. Administer by spoon or squeeze bottle, placing the slurry in the animal's cheek pouch.

Green Foods

Freshly minced wheat grass, wheat grass juice, powdered wheat grass and other cereal grasses, as well as green foods such as spirulina and chlorella, help prevent toxic reactions and rid the body of heavy metals, harmful chemicals, and other poisons. See pages 81–84.

Essential Oils

Many essential oils support detoxification and help the body's filtering organs and organs of elimination work more effectively. One of the simplest detoxification treatments is to place one drop of a blend of 2 to 3 parts lavender essential oil to 1 part peppermint oil on your dog's neck at the base of the skull, then place additional drops 2 to 4 inches apart down the spine and along the shoulder line. Substitute hydrosols for use on cats.

Dilute solutions of sage, thyme, eucalyptus, clary sage, and immortelle (*Helichrysum* species), as well as full-strength, therapeutic-grade sandalwood, chamomile, and rose oils also can be used on dogs. Hydrosols of these herbs are recommended for external use on cats.

Essential oils and hydrosols added to food, as described on pages 188–189, also support detoxification.

Appendix

Latin and Common Names of Popular Herbs

Achillea millefolium: yarrow

Agropyron repens: couch grass

alfalfa (*Medicago sativa*)

Allium sativum: garlic

aloe vera (*Aloe vera*)

Arctium lappa: burdock

arnica (*Arnica montana*)

Artemisia absinthium: wormwood

Artemisia annua: sweet Annie,
annual wormwood

Artemisia vulgaris: mugwort

ashwagandha (*Withenia somnifera*)

astragalus (*Astragalus membranaceous*)

Avena sativa: oats, oatstraw

bayberry (*Myrica cerifera*)

blackberry (*Rubus villosus, R. ursinus*)

black cohosh (*Cimicifuga racemosa*)

blue cohosh (*Caulophyllum
thalictroides*)

black walnut (*Juglans nigra*)

blue vervain (*Verbena hastata*)

boswellia (*Boswellia seratta*)

bupleurum (*Bupleurum* spp.)

burdock (*Arctium lappa*)

calendula (*Calendula officinalis*)

catnip (*Nepeta cataria*)

Caulophyllum thalictroides:
blue cohosh

Centella asiatica: gotu kola

chamomile (*Matricaria chamomilla,
Anthemia nobilis*)

chaparral (*Larrea tridentata*)

Cimicifuga racemosa: black cohosh

cleavers (*Galium aparine*)

clove (*Eugenia caryophyllata*)

coltsfoot (*Tussilago farfara*)

comfrey (*Symphytum officinale*)

Commiphora erythrea: myrrh, opopanax

Commiphora myrrha: myrrh, common

cornsilk (*Zea mays*)

couchgrass (*Agropyron repens*)

Crataegus oxyacantha: hawthorn berry

dandelion (*Taraxacum officinale*)

devil's claw root (*Harpagophytum
procumbens*)

echinacea (*Echinacea purpurea,
E. angustifolia*)

Eleutherococcus senticosus:
Siberian ginseng

Equisetum arvense: horsetail

Eugenia spp.: clove

feverfew (*Tanacetum parthenium*)

fo-ti (*Polygonum multiflorum*)

Galeum aparine: cleavers

garlic (*Allium sativum*)

gingerroot (*Zingiber officinale*)

ginkgo (*Ginkgo biloba*)

ginseng (*Panax ginseng, P. quinque-folius*)

Glycyrrhiza glabra, G. uralensis: licorice root

goldenseal (*Hydrastis canadensis*)

gotu kola (*Centella asiatica*)

Harpagophytum procumbens: devil's claw root

hawthorn berry (*Crataegus oxyacantha*)

hops (*Humulus lupulus*)

horsetail (*Equisetum arvense*)

Humulus lupulus: hops

Hydrastis canadensis: goldenseal

Hypericum perforatum: St. John's wort

Juglans nigra: black walnut

kava kava (*Piper methysticum*)

kelp (*Laminaria longicrucis*)

Laminaria longicrucis: kelp

Larrea tridentata: chaparral

Lavandula officinalis: lavender

lavender (*Lavandula officinalis, L. angustifolia, L. latifolia*)

licorice root (*Glycyrrhiza glabra, G. uralensis*)

lobelia (*Lobelia inflata*)

Matricaria chamomilla: chamomile

Medicago sativa: alfalfa

Melaleuca alternifolia: tea tree

Mentha piperita: peppermint

Mentha pulegium: pennyroyal

Mentha spicata: spearmint

milk thistle seed (*Silybum marianum*)

Morinda citrifolia: noni

mugwort (*Artemisia vulgaris*)

mullein (*Verbascum thepsus*)

Myrica cerifera: bayberry

myrrh, common (*Commiphora myrrha*)

myrrh, opopanax (*Commiphora erythraea*)

Nepeta cataria: catnip

nettle, stinging (*Urtica dioica*)

noni (*Morinda citrifolia*)

oats, oatstraw (*Avena sativa*)

Olea europaea: olive

olive (*Olea europaea*)

Panax ginseng, P. quinquefolius: ginseng

parsley (*Petroselinum sativum*)

Passiflora incarnata: passionflower

passionflower (*Passiflora incarnata*)

pau d'arco (*Tabebuia impetiginosa*)

pennyroyal (*Mentha pulegium*)

peppermint (*Mentha piperita*)

Petroselinum sativum: parsley

Piper methysticum: kava kava

Plantago psyllium: psyllium spp.

plantain (*Plantago* spp.)

Plantago (Eugenia Thynus): plantain

Polygonum multiflorum: fo-ti

psyllium (*Plantago psyllium*)

raspberry leaf (*Rubus idaeus*)

red clover (*Trifolium pratense*)

Rheum palmatum: Turkey rhubarb root

Rubus idaeus: raspberry leaf

Rubus villosus: blackberry

rue (*Ruta graveolens*)

Rumex acetosella: sheep sorrel

Ruta graveolens: rue

schisandra (*Schizandra chinensis*)

Schizandra chinensis: schisandra

Scutellaria laterifolia: skullcap

sheep sorrel (*Rumex acetosella*)

Siberian ginseng (*Eleutherococcus senticosus*)

Silybum marianum: milk thistle seed

skullcap (*Scutellaria laterifolia*)

slippery elm bark (*Ulmus fulva*)

spearmint (*Mentha spicata, M. aquitica*)

St. John's wort (*Hypericum perforatum*)

sweet Annie or annual wormwood (*Artemisia annua*)

Symphytum officinale: comfrey

Tabebuia impetiginosa: pau d'arco

Tanacetum parthenium: feverfew

Taraxacum officinale: dandelion

tea tree (*Melaleuca alternafolia*)

thyme (*Thymus* spp.)

Thymus spp: thyme

Trifolium pratense: red clover

Turkey rhubarb root (*Rheum palmatum*)

Tussilago farfara: coltsfoot

Ulmus fulva: slippery elm bark

Urtica dioica: nettle, stinging

valerian root (*Valeriana officinalis*)

Valeriana officinalis: valerian root

Verbascum thepsus: mullein

Verbena hastata: blue vervain

Withenia somnifera: ashwagandha

wormwood (*Artemisia absinthium*)

yarrow (*Achillea millefolium*)

yucca (*Yucca battaca*)

Yucca battaca: yucca

Zea mays: cornsilk

Zingiber officinale: gingerroot

Recommended Reading

de Bairacli Levy, Juliette. *The Complete Herbal Handbook for the Dog and Cat*. London: Faber and Faber. First published 1953; rev. ed. 1991.
———. *Cats Naturally*. London: Faber and Faber, 1991.
Belfield, Wendell O., and Martin Zucker. *How to Have a Healthier Dog*. New York: New American Library, 1981.
———. *The Very Healthy Cat Book*. San Jose, Calif.: Orthomolecular Specialties, 1983.
Billinghurst, Ian. *Give Your Dog a Bone*. Lithgow, N.S.W., Australia: Ian Billinghurst, 1993.
Buchman, Dian Dincin. *Herbal Medicine*. New York: Random House, 1996.
———. *Feed Your Pups with Bones*. Lithgow, N.S.W., Australia: Ian Billinghurst, 1998.
Clark, Hulda. *The Cure for All Diseases*. San Diego, Calif.: ProMotion Publishing, 1994.
Frazier, Anitra, and Norma Eckroate. *The New Natural Cat*. New York: Plume/Penguin Books, 1990.
Grosjean, Nelly. *Veterinary Aromatherapy*. Essex, England: C.W. Daniel Co., Ltd., 1994. Translated from the French by Joanne Robinson.
Lawless, Julia. *The Encyclopedia of Essential Oils*. Dorset, England, and Rockport, Mass.: Element Books Limited, 1992.
Ley, Beth M. *Dr. John Willard's Catalyst Altered Water*. Fargo, N.D.: Christopher Lawrence Communications, 1990.
Lust, John. *The Herb Book*. New York: Bantam Books, 1974. (Excellent, inexpensive basic herbal.)
McKay, Pat. *Reigning Cats and Dogs*. Pasadena, Calif.: Oscar Publications, 1996.
PDR for Herbal Medicines. Montvale, N.J.: Medical Economics Company, 1998. (Annual handbook from the *Physicians' Desk Reference* publisher. Very authoritative.)
Pitcairn, Richard, and Susan Hubble Pitcairn. *Natural Health for Dogs and Cats*. Emmaus, Penn.: Rodale Press, 1995.
Pottenger, Francis M., Jr. *Pottenger's Cats: A Study in Nutrition*. La Mesa, Calif.: Price-Pottenger Nutrition Foundation, 1983.

Puotinen, CJ. *The Encyclopedia of Natural Pet Care*. Los Angeles:
  Keats Publishing, 1998. (Companion to the book you are reading.)
Schultze, Kymythy R. *The Ultimate Diet: Natural Nutrition for Dogs and Cats*.
  Descanso, Calif.: Affenbar Ink, 1998.
Sheppard-Hanger, Sylla. *The Aromatherapy Practitioner Reference Manual*.
  Tampa, Fla.: Atlantic Institute of Aromatherapy, 1994. (Two-volume
  technical reference for aromatherapists and serious students.)
Stein, Diane. *The Natural Remedy Book for Dogs and Cats*. Freedom, Calif.:
  The Crossing Press, 1994.
Volhard, Wendy, and Kerry Brown. *The Holistic Guide for a Healthy Dog*.
  New York: Macmillan/Howell Book House, 1995.
Worwood, Valerie Ann. *The Complete Book of Essential Oils and
  Aromatherapy*. London: Macmillan London Limited, 1990; San Rafael,
  Calif.: New World Library, 1991.
Yarnall, Celeste. *Cat Care, Naturally*. Boston: Charles E. Tuttle Co., Inc.,
  1995.
———. *Natural Dog Care*. Boston: Charles E. Tuttle Co., Inc., 1998.

Resources

The following addresses, telephone and fax numbers, E-mail addresses, and Web site addresses are all subject to change. The reference librarian at your public library may be able to locate publishers and manufacturers that have moved since this book went to press. The area codes 800 and 888 are toll-free in the United States.

Books

Dog and Cat Book Catalog

Direct Book Service
P.O. Box 2778
Wenatchee, IA 98807-2778
1-800-776-2665 or 509-663-9115,
fax 509-662-7233
E-mail: dgctbook@cascade.net
www.dogandcatbooks.com

The most comprehensive dog and cat reference catalog imaginable.

Newsletters and Magazines

Alternatives

Mountain Home Publishing
1201 Seven Locks Rd.
Rockville, MD 20854
1-800-527-3044

Monthly newsletter edited by David G. Williams, M.D. Information often applies to dogs and cats.

Aromatic Thymes

P.O. Box 5041
Brentwood, TN 37024
847-304-0975, fax 847-304-0989
www.AromaticThymes.com

Quarterly aromatherapy magazine.

The Dog Love Letter

Animal Tales, LLC
P.O. Box 1855
North Falmouth, MA 02556-1855
Phone or fax 508-563-7162

Monthly newsletter edited by Beverly Cappel, D.V.M. Natural health and healing for dogs.

Country Living's Healthy Living
Hearst Communications, Inc.
959 Eighth Ave.
New York, NY 10019
1-800-925-0485

Bimonthly magazine of natural remedies, with occasional pet health articles.

Health Alert
P.O. Box 22620
Carmel, CA 93922-2620
408-372-2103

Edited by Bruce West, M.D. Monthly health newsletter for humans, with emphasis on whole-food supplements; information applies to dogs and cats.

The Herb Companion
Herb Companion Press
P.O. Box 55295
Boulder, CO 80322-5295
1-800-456-5835
www.Interweave.com

Bimonthly general-interest magazine.

The Herb Quarterly
Long Mountain Press, Inc.
223 San Anselmo Ave., Ste. 7
San Anselmo, CA 94960

Quarterly general-interest magazine, with occasional pet care articles.

HerbalGram
See American Botanical Council under Organizations.

Holistic Hound Newsletter
Marion Street Press, Inc.
P.O. Box 2249
Oak Park, IL 60303-2249
1-888-219-2509

Monthly newsletter of natural health for dogs.

Love of Animals
Earth Animal
P.O. Box 809
Wilton, CT 06897

Monthly newsletter of holistic pet care published by Susan and Robert Goldstein, D.V.M.

Natural Pet
This magazine is no longer published.

Natural Rearing
Marina Zacharias
P.O. Box 1436
Jacksonville, OR 97530
541-899-2080, fax 541-899-3414
E-mail: ambrican@cdsnet.net
www.naturalrearing.com

Newsletter of natural therapies for dogs and cats. Publishes annual directory of breeders who raise animals on a natural diet with few or no vaccinations.

Tiger Tribe
This magazine is no longer
published.

The Whole Cat Journal
P.O. Box 420031
Palm Coast, FL 32142-8624
1-800-829-9165
E-mail: customer_service@
belvoir.com

Monthly magazine of natural cat
care; no commercial advertising.

The Whole Dog Journal
Same publisher as *The Whole Cat
Journal*. Monthly 24-page magazine
of natural dog care and training; no
commercial advertising.

Organizations

**Academy of Veterinary
Homeopathy**
751 N.E. 168th St.
North Miami Beach, FL 33162
305-652-1590, fax 305-653-7244
www.theavh.org

Referrals to veterinary homeopaths.

American Botanical Council
P.O. Box 144345
Austin, TX 78714-4345
512-926-4900, fax 512-926-2345
E-mail: abc@herbalgram.org *or*
              custserve@herbalgram.org
www.herbalgram.org

Educational and research
organization, publisher of
HerbalGram, a quarterly magazine
devoted to herbal medicine.
Excellent resource.

American Herb Association
P.O. Box 1673
Nevada City, CA 95959
Phone/fax 916-274-3140

Educational organization, quarterly
newsletter.

American Herbalists Guild
P.O. Box 746555
Arvada, CO 80006-6555
303-423-8800, fax 303-428-8828

Professional organization, practitioners, referrals, quarterly newsletter.

**American Holistic Veterinary
Medical Association**
2218 Old Emmorton Rd.
Bel Air, MD 21015
410-569-0795, fax 410-569-2346
E-mail: ahvma@compuserve.com
www.altvedmed.com

Referrals to holistic veterinarians.

Herb Research Foundation
1007 Pearl St., Ste. 200
Boulder, CO 80302
303-449-2265, fax 303-449-7849
E-mail: info@herbs.org
www.herbs.org
Library of 100,000 scientific articles
on the safety and health benefits of
herbs. Excellent resource.

International Herb Association
P.O. Box 317
Mundelein, IL 60060
847-949-4372, fax 847-949-5896
E-mail: ihacathy@aol.com
Association of herb professionals.
Newsletter, activities.

National Association for Holistic Aromatherapy
P.O. Box 17622
Boulder, CO 80308
1-888-ASK-NAHA (1-888-275-6242)
www.naha.org

Northeast Herbal Association
P.O. Box 10
Newport, NY 13416
E-mail:
    NEHA@ www.jeansgreens.com
Educational, professional
organization; journal, activities.

The Pacific Institute of Aromatherapy
P.O. Box 6723
San Rafael, CA 94903
415-479-9121

United Plant Savers
P.O. Box 420
East Barre, VT 05549
802-479-9825, fax 802-476-3722
E-mail: ups@ilhawaii.net
Nonprofit, grassroots organization
for the restoration and cultivation
of environmentally threatened
medicinal plants.

Foods and Nutritional Supplements

Advanced Nutrition Products
P.O. Box 1634
Rockville, MD 20850
1-888-436-7200, fax 301-963-3886
ImmunoGuard brand lactoferrin,
Oralmat rye grass extract.

Alternative Treatment Information Network, Inc.
1582 W. Deere Ave., Ste. C
Irvine, CA 92606
1-800-446-3063
Immutol brand Beta 1, 3 D Glucan.

Ameriflex, Inc.
232 NE Lincoln St., Ste. G
Hillsboro, OR 97124
1-800-487-5463 or 503-640-0810
MinerAll 72, a liquid colloidal trace mineral supplement.

Amyx Naturals
363 Carroll Close
Tarrytown, NY 10591
1-800-395-7134 or 914-631-7788,
fax 914-524-9735
E-mail: petherbs@aol.com
Information about raw-meat suppliers for pets.

Animal Food Services, Inc.
675 E. State St.
Iola, WI 54945
1-800-743-0322, fax 715-445-4309
www.animalfood.com
Frozen raw-meat diets for zoo animals and domestic pets.

Bioforce of America
P.O. Box 507
Kinderhook, NY 12106
518-758-6060
Imports Biostrath and Animastrath liquid yeast from Switzerland; superior products.

Bio-Nutritional Formulas
106 E. Jericho Turnpike
P.O. Box 311
Mineola, NY 11501-0311
1-800-950-8484, fax 1-800-321-2573
Supplements, including thymic protein.

Cat's Claws, Inc.
1004 W. Broadway
Morrilton, AR 72110
1-800-783-0977 or 501-354-5015,
fax 501-354-4843
Cat products, including dehydrated tuna flakes (Tuna Dash) to flavor any food or tea for cats or dogs.

Eden Foods
701 Tecumseh Rd.
Clinton, MI 49236
1-800-248-0301 or 517-456-7424,
fax 517-456-6075
Imports sun-dried unrefined sea salt from northern France for sale in health food stores.

Gardens Alive
8100 Schenley Place
Lawrenceburg, IN 47025
812-537-8650, fax 812-537-5108
E-mail: gardener@gardensalive.com
Organic gardening supplies.

Gold Mine Natural Food Company
3419 Hancock St.
San Diego, CA 92110-4307
1-800-475-FOOD, fax 619-296-9756

Unrefined sea salt, Japanese salad presses, organic grains.

Golden Health Products, Inc.
6 Kentucky Rd.
Quincy, IL 62301
1-800-780-1198

Seacure and other supplements.

Grain and Salt Society
273 Fairway Drive
Asheville, NC 28805
1-800-867-7258 or 704-299-9005, fax 704-299-1640

Imports Celtic unrefined sea salt from France.

Hawks Hunt Farm
234 Gabryszewski Rd.
St. Johnsville, NY 13452-2316
1-800-7-FLY-DOG or 518-568-3325

Source of organically raised beef, chicken, turkey, and eggs for pets and people.

Healing Within Products, Inc.
84 Berkeley Ave.
San Anselmo, CA 94960
1-800-300-7548 or 415-454-6677, fax 415-454-6659

Supplements, informative catalog.

Holistic Pet Center
P.O. Box 1166
Clackamas, OR 97015
503-656-5342 or 1-800-788-PETS

Holistic pet supplies.

Immune Systems Products
5 Harris Court N6
Monterey, CA 93940
408-372-3805 or 1-800-231-8063

Standard Process supplements; catalog includes product descriptions.

International Yogurt Company
628 N. Doheny Drive
Los Angeles, CA 90069

Supplies health food stores with kefir grains, yogurt starter, and yogurt supplements.

Jaffee Bros. Natural Foods
P.O. Box 636
Valley Center, CA 92082
760-749-1133, fax 760-749-1282

Raw carob powder, organically grown nuts and dried fruits. Excellent quality.

Life Enhancement Products, Inc.
266 Saginaw Rd.
Sanford, MI 48657
1-800-914-6311

Seacure and other supplements.

Life Enhancement Products, Inc.

P.O. Box 751390
Petaluma, CA 94975-1390
1-800-543-3873 or 707-762-6144,
fax 707-769-8016
www.life-enhancement.com

Dr. Jonathan Wright's ThyroPlex
thyroid supplement and other
products.

Live Food Products

P.O. Box 7
Santa Barbara, CA 93102
1-800-446-1990
www.bragg.com

Manufactures raw, unfiltered,
unpasteurized Bragg Organic Apple
Cider Vinegar, sold in health food
stores and by mail order.

Merritt Naturals

P.O. Box 532
Rumson, NJ 07760
1-888-463-7748 or 732-530-7961

Herbal vitamins and essential fatty
acid supplements for dogs and cats.

Mezotrace Corporation

415 Wellington St.
Winnemucca, NV 89445-2666
1-800-843-9989 or 702-623-1151,
fax 702-623-1153

Powdered trace minerals for pets
and people.

Natural Lifestyle Supply Company

16 Lookout Drive
Asheville, NC 28804
1-800-292-4443

Organic seeds, grains, Japanese salad
presses.

Natural Pet Care

8050 Lake City Way
Seattle, WA 98115
1-800-962-8266 or 206-522-1667,
fax 206-522-1132
E-mail: petcare@halcyon.com
www.halcyon.com/petcare/

Catalog of recommended pet
supplies.

New Chapter, Inc.

22 High St.
P.O. Box 1947
Brattleboro, VT 05304
1-800-543-7279 or 802-257-0018,
fax 1-800-470-0247 or 802-257-0652
E-mail: zingiber@sover.net

Medicinal mushroom products,
nutritional supplements.

New England Cheesemaking Supply Company

P.O. Box 65
Ashfield, MA 01330
413-628-3808

Kefir culture, Bulgarian yogurt
culture, and several cheese starter
cultures.

North Star Natural Pet Products
RR1, Box 428B
Tinmouth, VT 05773
802-446-2812

Natural pet care products, herbs, books.

Nutrition Coalition
P.O. Box 8023
Fargo, ND 58109-8023
1-800-447-4793 or 701-235-4064

Willard Water extract, colostrum supplements.

Pat McKay, Inc.
396 W. Washington Blvd., Ste. 600
Pasadena, CA 91103
1-800-975-7555 or 626-296-1120,
fax 626-296-1126
E-mail: patmckay@gte.net
www.home1.gte.net/patmckay

Frozen raw foods, nutritional supplements, books.

PetNutrition
577 Humbolt
Denver, CO 80218
1-800-494-2659

Freeze-dried or frozen raw meats, enzymes, food-source vitamin/mineral supplements.

Pet's Friend, Inc.
7154 N. University Drive, Ste. 720
Tamarac, FL 33321
1-800-868-1009 or 954-720-0978,
fax 954-720-0978
E-mail: petsfriend@zim.com

Glandular concentrates, digestive enzymes, trace minerals.

Pet Sage
4313 Wheeler Ave.
Alexandria, VA 22304
1-800-PET-HLTH or 703-823-9711,
fax 703-823-9714
E-mail: info@petsage.com
www.petsage.com

Books, supplements, pet health products.

Preventive Therapies, Inc.
P.O. Box 956248
Duluth, GA 30096
1-800-556-5530 or 770-409-0900

Thymic supplements.

Prozyme Products, Ltd.
6600 N. Lincoln Ave., #312
Lincolnwood, IL 60645-3633
1-800-522- 5537, fax 847-982-1310

Prozyme enzyme powder.

Shiloh Farms
P.O. Box 97
Sulphur Springs, AR 72768

Health food store products, including raw carob powder.

Solid Gold Health Products for Pets
1483 N. Cuyamaca
El Cajon, CA 92020
619-258-1914

Buckaroo Beef, freeze-dried raw beef from free-range cattle.

Springtime, Inc.
10942-J Beaver Dam Rd.
P.O. Box 1227
Cockeysville, MD 21030
1-800-521-3212 or 410-771-8430, fax 410-771-1530

Natural supplements and food concentrates for dogs, horses, and people.

Standard Process, Inc.
1200 W. Royal Lee Drive
Palmyra, WI 53156
1-800-848-5061 or 414-495-2122, fax 414-495-2512

Product information for licensed health care professionals, not retail customers. Vitamin, mineral, glandular, and food supplement products from organically grown whole-food sources. Ask your holistic veterinarian for product recommendations (veterinary protocols brochure can be obtained from the manufacturer). Products available at some health food stores and mail-order companies, including the Vitamin Shoppe, Ambrican Enterprises, and Immune Systems Products (see separate listings). Immune Systems Products publishes a description of 56 Standard Process products and their uses.

Steve's Real Food for Dogs
3070 McKendrick Street
Eugene, OR 97405
1-888-526-1900 or 541-683-9950, fax 541-683-2035

Superior-quality frozen and freeze-dried fresh foods for dogs.

T.J. Clark & Company
1145 N. 1100 St. West
St. George, UT 84770
1-800-228-0872 or 801-634-0309, fax 801-634-0308

Liquid colloidal trace minerals.

Twenty-First Century Products
P.O. Box 562
Mineral Wells, TX 76068
940-325-9284, fax 940-328-1439

Panteric and Panteric Extra are pancreas gland peptone supplements for pets.

Veterinary Nutrition Corp.
522 E. Idaho Ave.
Las Cruces, NM 88001-3742
1-888-777-0505
www.balancediet.com

Manufactures BalanceDiet dog and cat foods made of high-quality ingredients, naturally preserved by fermentation.

The Vitamin Shoppe, Inc.
4700 Westside Ave.
North Bergen, NJ 07047
1-800-223-1216 or 201-866-7711,
fax 1-800-852-7153

Books, herbs, and supplements,
including Standard Process products, (although they are not listed in
the Vitamin Shoppe catalog).

Whiskers Holistic Pet Products
235 E. 9th St.
New York, NY 10003
1-800-WHISKERS or 212-979-2532,
fax 212-979-0075
E-mail: healthypet@msn.com
www.choicemall.com/whiskers

Frozen and fresh raw foods, books,
herbs, natural remedies.

Willner Chemists
100 Park Ave.
New York, NY 10017
1-800-633-1106 or 212-682-2817,
fax 212-682-6192

Supplements by mail order.

Wysong Institute
1880 N. Eastman Rd.
Midland, MI 48642-7779
517-631-0009, fax 517-631-8801
E-mail: wysong@tm.net

Natural supplements, pet nutrition
information, enzyme supplements.

Celeste Yarnall, Ph.D.
9875 Gloucester Dr.
Beverly Hills, CA 90210
1-888-CEL-PETS or 310-278-1385,
fax 310-278-3499
E-mail: Celeste@celestialpets.com
www.celestialpets.com

Fresh and frozen raw food,
supplements.

Herbs and Herbal Products

Ambrican Enterprises, Ltd.
Marina Zacharias
P.O. Box 1436
Jacksonville, OR 97530
541-899-2080, fax 541-899-3414
E-mail: ambrican@cdsnet.net

Natural supplements, herbs,
supplies. Importer of Juliette de
Bairacli Levy's Natural Rearing
herbal products for dogs and cats.

Amyx Naturals
363 Carroll Close
Tarrytown, NY 10591
1-800-395-7134 or 914-631-7788,
fax 914-524-9735
E-mail: petherbs@aol.com

Herbs and essential oils. Owner
Robin Amyx recommends Planet
Solution, a nontoxic cleaning
solution made of seed-bearing

plants, for hot spots, skin rashes, ringworm, and ear fungus as well as household cleaning. My source for amaranth oil.

Animal Friends International Mfg. Co.
P.O. Box 986
Abingdon, MD 21009
1-800-772-2559, fax 410-836-7305
E-mail: absonat@flash.net
www.absolutelynatural.com

Fast-acting stain and odor removers for home and kennel use (including skunk sprays and kennel runs), dog shampoos, conditioners, and grooming aids made of enzymes and beneficial bacteria. Recommended for pets and show dogs.

Avena Botanicals
P.O. Box 365
West Rockport, ME 04865
207-594-0694

Herbs, supplies. Grows and manufactures herbs for pets. Highly recommended.

Bea Lydecker's Naturals, Inc.
15443 S. Latourette Rd.
Oregon City, OR 97045
503-631-8589 or 503-631-7389

Herbs and natural supplements, including superior-quality Hawaiian noni powder.

Boston Jojoba Company
P.O. Box 771
Middleton, MA 01949
1-800-256-5622, fax 978-777-9332
E-mail: jojobabob@aol.com
Jojoba oil.

Casa Verde
817 Chestnut Ridge Rd.
Chestnut Ridge, NY 10977
914-352-2510, fax 914-352-2528
E-mail: casaverdeherb@juno.com
Superior-quality herbs, books, gifts.

Clover International
4420 S. Arville, #35
Las Vegas, NV 89103-3746
702-251-8880, fax 702-251-8288
www.livingfit.com
Chlorella powder by mail order.

CompassioNet
P.O. Box 710
Saddle River, NJ 07458-0710
1-800-510-2010 or 201-236-3900,
fax 201-236-0090
www.compassionet.com

Source of MGN-3, an immune-supporting supplement made from rice bran and medicinal mushroom extracts. Recommended for cancer prevention and treatment.

East Earth Trade Winds

P.O. Box 493151
1620 E. Cypress Ave., #8
Redding, CA 96049-3151
1-800-258-6878
www.snowcrest.net/eetw/

Traditional Chinese herbs.

East Park Research, Inc.

P.O. Box 530099
Henderson, NV 89053-0099
702-837-1111, fax 702-837-1110

Superior-quality olive leaf extract.

Frontier Cooperative Herbs

P.O. Box 299
Norway, IA 52318
1-800-669-3275
www.frontiercoop.com

Large wholesale/retail herb company. Empty gelatin capsules in large and very small sizes.

Gourmet & Mushroom Products

P.O. Box 515
Graton, CA 95444
1-800-789-9121 or 707-829-7301,
fax 707-823-9091
www.gmushrooms.com or
www.health.pon.net

Medicinal mushroom growing kits, mushroom extracts.

Herbal Science International, Inc.

1015 S. Nogales St.
Rowland Heights, CA 91748
626-965-0906

Superior-quality Chinese herbal products, including *Hsiao Chai Hu Tang*, a bupleurum formula for liver support.

Herb Pharm

P.O. Box 116
Williams, OR 97544
1-800-348-4372 or 1-800-599-2392,
fax 1-800-545-7392

Source of alkaloid-free comfrey, arnica tincture, and other superior-quality herbs.

Imhotep, Inc.

P.O. Box 183
Ruby, NY 12475
1-800-677-8577 or 914-336-2070

Manufactures ProSeed grapefruit seed extract liquid, capsules, ear wash, and other products.

Island Herbs

Ryan Drum
Waldron Island, WA 98297

Famous for seaweeds.

Jean's Greens

119 Sulphur Springs Rd.
Newport, NY 13416
1-888-845-TEAS or 315-845-6500

Herbs, supplies, books, free reports on herbal topics. Superior quality, inexpensive Essiac tea (brand name Forticell).

Karadsheh's Spice Bazaar, Inc.

3052 N. 16th St.
Phoenix, AZ 85016
1-800-307-7423, fax 602-277-0809
www.spicebazaar.com

Mastic gum, myrrh gum, and other spices.

Larreacorp, Ltd.

P.O. Box 6598
Chandler, AZ 85226
1-800-682-9448, fax 602-963-7310

Larreastat chaparral extract, treated to remove potential toxins.

Meadowbrook Herb Garden

93 Kingstown Rd.
Wyoming, RI 02898
1-888-539-7603

Biodynamically grown (a step beyond organic) medicinal teas. Superior quality, highly recommended.

Norimoor Company, Inc.

La Maison Francaise
5222 Fifth Avenue
New York, NY 10185-0043
212-695-MOOR or 212-268-5399,
fax 212-695-4535

Herbal Melange from Austria.

North American Tree Resin Company, Inc. (NATR)

2806 Broadway, Ste. 2
Eureka, CA 95501
1-800-422-4716 or 707-442-4716

Source of Native American tree resin (pitch) and olive oil ointments containing pitch. Pitch is a natural preservative and disinfectant.

Nuherbs Co.

3820 Penniman Ave.
Oakland, CA 94619
1-800-233-4307 or 510-534-4384,
fax 1-800-550-1928 or 510-534-4384

Superior-quality Chinese herbs.

Nutri-Biotic

P.O. Box 238
Lakeport, CA 95453
1-800-225-4345 or 707-263-0411,
fax 707-263-7844
E-mail: nutribio@pacific.net

Nutri-Biotic grapefruit seed extract liquid, capsules, tablets, nasal spray, ear drops, herbal insect repellent, and other products.

Pines International, Inc.
P.O. Box 1107
Lawrence, KS 66044-8107
1-800-697-4637 or 913-841-6016,
fax 913-841-1252

Superior-quality wheat grass and
other grass powders and tablets.
Rhubarb powder.

Richters
357 Highway 47
Goodwood, Ontario
Canada L0C 1A0
905-640-6677, fax 905-640-6641
E-mail: orderdesk@richters.com

Outstanding free catalog of herb
plants and seeds, excellent shipping
service, superior quality; also sells
dried herbs and books. With its pho-
tographs and concise descriptions of
several hundred herbs, the catalog
doubles as an herb reference book.

Robert McDowell, Herbalist
Bathurst Traditional Medicine Centre
221 George St.
Bathurst, New South Wales, 2795
Australia
011-61-063-313937,
fax 011-61-063-324494
E-mail: Robert.McDowell@
    herbal-treatments.com.au
www.herbal-treatments.com.au

Herbal formulas for pets, including
the equisetum (horsetail) tincture for
bone cancer described on page 150.

Root to Health
P.O. Box 509
Wausau, WI 54402-0509
1-800-388-3818 or 715-675-2326,
fax 715-675-9730
E-mail: info@hsuginseng.com

Hsu's Ginseng. Excellent quality,
informative catalog.

Sage Mountain Herb Products
P.O. Box 420
East Barre, VT 05649
802-479-9825

Rosemary Gladstar's herbal products
company. Recommended.

Simplers Botanicals
P.O. Box 39
Forestville, CA 95436
707-887-2012, fax 707-887-8570

James Green's herbal products
company. Recommended.

The Sprout House
17267 Sundance Drive
Ramona, CA 92065
1-800-SPROUTS
E-mail: info@SproutHouse.com
www.SproutHouse.com

Seeds, supplies, and information
about sprouting.

Tasha's Herbs

P.O. Box 9888
Jackson, WY 83002
1-800-315-0142, fax 307-734-0144
E-mail: tashaherbs@wyoming.com

Herbal products for dogs and cats.
Recommended.

Therapeutic Botanicals, Inc.

2711 NW Sixth St., Ste. B
Gainesville, FL 32609
1-877-890-6336 (toll-free)
or 352-381-9496, fax 352-375-2663

Grows neem organically in Mexico,
imports and manufactures neem
products, including seed oil, extract,
leaf, powder, and skin cream.
Detailed instructions for using neem
with dogs available online at:
www.neemaura.com/Misc/dogs_and_
    neem.htm.

TransPacific Health Products

3924 Central Ave.
St. Petersburg, FL 33711
1-800-336-9636

Traditional Chinese herbs.

Essential Oils and Aromatherapy Products

`Acqua Vita

85 Arundel Ave.
Toronto, Ontario
Canada M4K 3A3
416-405-8855
E-mail: acquavita@interlog.com

Essential oils, hydrosols, and a therapeutic wall chart showing the known
and experimental properties of 40
aromatic distillates (hydrosols) and
their applications. Suzanne Catty's
aromatherapy products company.
Recommended.

Aromaleigh, Inc.

180 St. Paul St. #402
Rochester, NY 14604
1-877-894-2283 (toll-free)
www.aromaleigh.com

Aromatherapy products for dogs,
cats, and people from Kristen Leigh
Bell. Recommended.

Aromatherapy International

150 Staniford St., Ste. 632
Boston, MA 02114
1-800-722-4377 or 617-670-1792,
fax 617-846-0285
E-mail: eurolink@umich.edu

Distributes essential oils and
hydrosols grown and distilled by
Nelly Grosjean, author of *Veterinary
Aromatherapy*. Recommended.

JPT Aromatherapy
1901 Brule St.
South Lake Tahoe, CA 96150
1-888-278-7364 or 530-577-5338,
fax 530-577-5722
E-mail: jptaroma@thetahoe.net

The world's largest line of authentic
wild and organic essential oils,
including 50 hydrosols.
Recommended.

Liberty Natural Products
8120 SE Stark St.
Portland, OR 98714-2356
1-800-289-8427, fax 503-256-1182
E-mail: Liberty@teleport.com

www.teleport.com/~liberty

Essential oils, books, supplies. My
source of opopanax essential oil and
water-soluble sulfated castor oil.

Scents of Smell
P.O. Box 182
Derby, CT 06418
1-888-389-0060

Aromatherapy products for dogs
and cats from Patricia Whitaker.
Recommended.

Index